Understanding Doulas and Childbirth

Cheryl A. Hunter • Abby Hurst

Understanding Doulas and Childbirth

Women, Love, and Advocacy

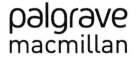

Cheryl A. Hunter
University of North Dakota
Grand Forks, North Dakota, USA

Abby Hurst
Ph.D. candidate
A.T. Still University
Allen, Texas, USA

ISBN 978-1-137-48535-9   ISBN 978-1-137-48536-6   (eBook)
DOI 10.1057/978-1-137-48536-6

Library of Congress Control Number: 2016938702

© The Editor(s) (if applicable) and The Author(s) 2016
This work is subject to copyright. All rights are solely and exclusively licensed by the Publisher, whether the whole or part of the material is concerned, specifically the rights of translation, reprinting, reuse of illustrations, recitation, broadcasting, reproduction on microfilms or in any other physical way, and transmission or information storage and retrieval, electronic adaptation, computer software, or by similar or dissimilar methodology now known or hereafter developed.
The use of general descriptive names, registered names, trademarks, service marks, etc. in this publication does not imply, even in the absence of a specific statement, that such names are exempt from the relevant protective laws and regulations and therefore free for general use.
The publisher, the authors and the editors are safe to assume that the advice and information in this book are believed to be true and accurate at the date of publication. Neither the publisher nor the authors or the editors give a warranty, express or implied, with respect to the material contained herein or for any errors or omissions that may have been made. The publisher remains neutral with regard to jurisdictional claims in published maps and institutional affiliations.

Cover illustration: © Blend Images / Alamy Stock Photo

Printed on acid-free paper

This Palgrave Macmillan imprint is published by Springer Nature
The registered company is Nature America Inc. New York

To my devoted and often roguish dissertation doula, for with him everything in my life is possible. To Aislinn and Ceallan, this project is for you. Your births ignited my passions: a passion for knowledge, a passion for equity, a passion to be grounded in the feminine.

Much gratitude goes to my dedicated committee who understood and supported my commitment to social justice and concern for women and children in birth. Their intellect and patience helped support the birth of this research project. Barbara, Bradley, Donna, and Luise—you will continue to serve as guides reflecting academic intellect, honesty, and care.

To the wonderful Powerfrau, with whose support and words of wisdom in the most difficult of times, I have persevered.

To Georg'ann, who saw our youngest come into this world and since then has continued to be one of my greatest role models.

To the doulas and birthing women who contributed their insights on birth, their time, and their wonderful energy—I am forever in their debt.
Cheryl Hunter

To Izzy, Maxwell, and Jackson—thank you for letting me be your mom. Every day is better because of you. To Greg, thank you for being my Favorite Person. Sorry there are no dragons in this book, I tried.

Many thanks to the mothers, fathers, and doulas who volunteered their time and shared personal stories. It was very moving to have so many people share intimate and emotional details in order to make this book possible. And, of course, Cheryl—thank you for allowing me to join you on this awesome journey! I will be forever grateful to you for this experience.
Abby Hurst

Contents

1 Childbirth, Women, and Doulas 1

2 Nurses, Families, and Doulas: An Overview of Different Roles in Childbirth 25

3 Alienation and a Challenge to Authority in Childbirth 51

4 Birthing with Doulas: The Embodied Birth Experience 73

5 Love and Advocacy in Childbirth 99

References 125

Index 137

About the Authors

Cheryl Hunter Ph.D. As a sociologist of teaching and learning my primary focus is on microlevel analyses: educational interactions that happen between individuals and the different intercultural contexts in which those interactions arise. I consider myself a *translational researcher*, producing research that reaches the people for whom it is intended in a practical way and in a way which contributes to improving their life experiences or professional practice. I have extensive experience in a wide range of qualitative methodologies. I received both a Spencer Fellowship at Indiana University and a post-doctoral research fellowship at Cleveland Clinic College of Medicine, giving me wide-ranging experiences in phenomenology, content analysis, grounded theory, cognitive task analysis, and critical ethnography.

Abby Hurst M.S. As a health care clinician, my focus has always been on science, and how science can improve our life experiences and expectancy. As I progressed through my career, I began to realize that my patients needed more than the practical knowledge science provides; they needed an advocate who could empower them to take back control of their health. Through my professional development and academic studies, I slowly transitioned away from being a clinician to being a patient advocate. I now work with patients, guiding and educating them on how to have productive conversations with their health care team. My current doctoral research focuses on interprofessional communication between doulas and hospital-based maternity care providers.

CHAPTER 1

Childbirth, Women, and Doulas

> *The other day I was finally able to write down my thoughts and memories in a journal. Writing it all down helped me realize how much the labor transformed me as an individual. I was able to find strength deep within myself that I never knew I had. Thank you. (Amy, mother)*

This note of thanks written to Amy's labor support woman, referred to as her doula, displays the intensity with which some women view the childbirth with a doula and the birthing experience itself as transformative. While not every birthing woman has the same experience with a doula, the overall medical consensus is that doulas provide positive childbirth outcomes for women and their babies. One of the roles of the doula, specifically in hospital childbirth, is to advocate for the laboring woman as she navigates the medical system in addition to providing continuous physical and emotional support. How and in what way this happens is the target of this book. This research investigated the work of doulas and the perceptions of how doulas differed from other medical personnel. It examined the different aspects of the doulas' role as they prepared, accompanied, and then reflected back with the birthing woman and her partner about the childbirth experience.

This book offers several critiques. Firstly, it critiques the medical institutional model for asserting that medical knowledge, specifically through the use of technology and interventions, is *the only* valid knowledge about childbirth, and as a result, women in childbirth no longer possess any authority to define their own knowledge as "expertise." The institutionalized structures of power that define *what* knowledge is and *who* can possess it (Code 1991, p. 177) impose an external authority upon women, relegating women's bodily knowledge as, at best, inferior or simply as nonexistent. Secondly, the female body has been portrayed as pathological and deficient, requiring external intervention during childbirth for all women, not just those with risk factors. In contrast, the doula views women's bodies as inherently capable and resilient in childbirth, and that normal birth requires no need for intervention. The doula also focuses on the experience of birth, and views it as something transformative and to be privileged. Likewise, the doula-led experience is centered on the woman's body in an active role in the childbirth process, creating an *embodied* experience. Lastly, doulas model to their clients both love and advocacy because doulas believe that modeling these behaviors will translate as women become mothers through the process of childbirth.

Defining the Role of the Doula

According to Doulas of North America International (DONA), one of the largest doula training and advocacy organizations in the USA, doulas are trained and experienced in childbirth to provide women and their partners physical, emotional, and informational support during labor and birth (DONA 2005). Doula is a Greek word meaning "woman servant," (ICEA Position Paper 1999). Historically, laboring women have turned to other women for help and support during the laboring process (Ashford 1998; Wertz and Wertz 1989; Barry and Paxson 1971). The progression from a labor support woman with personal birth experience to a paraprofessional woman trained in childbirth education and labor support techniques has led the recent generation of labor support women to carve a newly legitimized social role for themselves, being referred to as doulas.

The doula offers help and advice on comfort measures, such as breathing, relaxation, movement, and positioning. She also assists families in gathering information about the course of their labor and their options. Doulas specialize in nonmedical skills and do not perform clinical tasks, such as vaginal exams or fetal heart rate monitoring. Doulas do not diagnose or give medical advice. An important distinction to make is that the role of the doula is not to interfere with the roles of other labor support staff, or provide a dissenting opinion to what the medical staff is recommending.

According to advocacy literature, the doula's goal is to help the birthing woman have a safe and satisfying childbirth as the woman concerned defines it, which results in a multiplicity of outcomes such as decreased use of analgesics, fewer complications during labor, and higher initiation rates of breast-feeding (Gruber et al. 2013). It has been noted that when a doula was present, some women felt reduced need for pain medications, or postponed them until later in labor; however, many women chose or needed pharmacological pain relief (DONA 2005). Doulas do not offer opinions or voice disapproval of decisions the laboring woman makes (Gilliland 2011; Meyer et al. 2001). The doulas' role as educator is defined as helping women become informed about various options, including the risks, benefits, and accompanying precautions or interventions for safety (Gurevich 2003). The doula provides information about normal birthing processes and medical options available during the birth. The doula demonstrates to family members and friends how to help the mother be more comfortable and how to play a useful role in her labor and delivery (DONA 2005). A doula can provide suggestions to the partner as to what comfort measures may help the birthing mother. Doulas can also work with the birth partner in order to relieve any stress of the partner so that he/she is fully able to participate in the birth process (Bäckström and Hertfelt Wahn 2011).

Therefore, the doula has been identified as performing three overarching roles: physical and emotional support, education, and advocacy (DONA 2005). Physical and emotional support can include providing a constant, supportive presence and empowering the woman to ask questions. Doulas also provide nonjudgmental support and education, allowing for informed decision-making by the mother and partner (Amram et al. 2014). Doulas, in advocating for the laboring woman, "facilitate positive communication between provider and client, helping both partners and providers address and consider the woman's fears" (Pascali-Bonaro 2003, p. 5).

Why might women need a doula during childbirth? The notion of an external advocate brought into the hospital may reflect the "alien environment" of the hospital where "women need someone to explain medical jargon or express her wishes to the clinicians" (Madi et al. 1999, p. 5). The doula provides a fundamentally different service than clinical health care professionals in the hospital setting. Doulas traditionally served women in the homebirth setting until their recent professionalization and organization, which promoted their role in hospital births (Morton 2002). The role of the doula is not well-defined in many health care facilities, and as such, many health care providers do not fully understand the role of the doula within the facility. Health care providers may even believe the doula is there to oppose any medical intervention. The narratives in this book support the belief that doulas often question the high rates of medical interventions in childbirth, fundamentally lodging a critique about the medicalization of childbirth.

THE MEDICALIZATION OF AMERICAN BIRTHING PRACTICES

Pregnancy and childbirth were once considered an exclusively female domain. Women who were in labor would rarely give birth in a hospital setting, choosing instead to deliver at home, with the support of other women assisting with the labor. Women attended to each other during labor and weeks of postpartum recovery. Medical intervention was rare. It was not until the late 1700s that medical doctors began attending childbirth (Wertz and Wertz 1989). The idea that childbirth is a natural process and not a medical procedure remained popular in the USA until the 1920s. Up until that time, less than 5 % of childbirths took place in a hospital (Wertz and Wertz 1989). After the 1920s there was a drastic shift toward the medicalization of childbirth. It is estimated that by the mid-1950s, almost 95 % of childbirths took place within a hospital (van Teijlingen et al. 2009). By this time, labor was no longer thought of as a natural process that occurs without the need for medical intervention, but instead, a procedure that requires input and monitoring from physicians and nurses. Today women rarely choose to give birth at home with only the support of other women. Now, women are being taught the potential risks of childbirth and encouraged to accept the medicalized nature of childbirth (Chmell 2012).

Conrad (1992) defined medicalization as "a process by which non-medical problems become defined and treated as medical conditions, usually in terms of illnesses or disorder" (p. 210). The medicalization of childbirth caused a paradigm shift in the way society viewed the need for medical intervention. Childbirth has been redefined as a dangerous event that women are incapable of handling without the support of physicians and other clinical staff. Obstetricians and other clinical staff have taken over the responsibility of aiding women even during uncomplicated labor. This is being done despite the recommendation that medical interventions should occur only if "they are of benefit to the woman or her baby"

(Department of Health 2004, p. 4). Often women with uncomplicated pregnancies are encouraged to use epidural analgesics, fetal monitoring, and other medical interventions with no documented outcome to the mother or baby (Johanson et al. 2002).

MEDICAL INTERVENTIONS USED ON WOMEN IN CHILDBIRTH

Some of the more common medical interventions during labor include induction of labor, electronic fetal monitoring (EFM), episiotomies, and cesarean sections (c-sections). Physicians may recommend medical interventions due to either the baby or the mother being in distress, or to speed up the process of labor for the convenience of either the medical staff or the patient.

Elective Induction

Elective induction involves artificially stimulating the uterus to initiate labor. Typically this is performed by either rupturing the amniotic membranes or administering Pitocin. Pitocin is a synthetic version of oxytocin—the naturally produced hormone that stimulates uterine contractions and lactation. With noninduced labor, oxytocin allows for more regulated contractions as it is secreted in bursts, rather than continuously. Pitocin, conversely, is administered in a steady intravenous flow, thus leading to more powerful and faster contractions. The stronger Pitocin-induced contractions may lead to a decrease in uterine blood flow, possibly decreasing oxygen to the fetus (WHO 2011). The stronger contractions and decrease in oxygen to the fetus also necessitate the use of EFM.

Additionally, unlike oxytocin, Pitocin does not cross the blood–brain barrier. When oxytocin circulates through the blood–brain barrier, it causes the release of endorphins. Endorphins work on the same receptors in the brain as do chemical opiates, providing pain relief. In addition to this, they can also induce feelings of euphoria. Therefore, without crossing the blood–brain barrier, a Pitocin-induced labor is unlikely to provide the same natural pain relief (Lothian 2006). Thus, in order to provide pain relief during an induced labor, an epidural or other analgesic must be administered, consequently leading to a cascade of additional medical interventions.

Electronic Fetal Monitoring (EFM)

Electronic fetal monitoring (EFM) is a common medical intervention used during pregnancy. It is used in order to evaluate the uterine contractions of the mother and subsequent heart rate of the fetus. EFM was developed in order to provide a way to monitor the fetus for any signs of crisis and subsequent need for a quick delivery. The impetus for the development of this technology was to reduce the rate of cerebral palsy and mental retardation caused by insufficient oxygen flow to the baby during labor and resultant hypoxia (ACOG 2009) as physicians could intervene at the first signs of abnormal heart rate patterns.

EFM requires the woman to be attached to electronic bands and monitors; this can decrease the comfort of the woman by limiting her ability to ambulate. Even portable monitors have been shown to be cumbersome and limit the movements of laboring women (Jansen et al. 2013). More importantly, EFM has been shown to have a very high rate of false positive readings, leading to an increase in unnecessary forceps-assisted births and c-sections. Randomized clinical trials have shown that EFM has little benefit over listening to the fetal heart rate by using an external acoustical device with regard to mortality or neurological outcomes (Thacker et al. 1995). As far back as 1989, the American Congress of Obstetricians and Gynecologists (ACOG) issued a policy statement offering intermittent auscultation for low-risk pregnant women as an alternative to EFM (ACOG 2009).

Episiotomy

Episiotomy is a surgical incision made around the perineum. It was once thought that the proactive surgical incision would prevent more extensive tears that would have formed naturally during delivery. However, many hospitals continue to perform routine episiotomies, regardless of medical need, in order to decrease time spent pushing during delivery. In a normally progressing labor, with no signs of fetal distress, routine episiotomies have not been shown to benefit mother and baby. Episiotomies have been shown to increase the risk of pain, infection, urinary and fecal incontinence, and sexual dysfunction in the mother (ACOG 2006). Hartmann et al. (2005) studied the effects routine episiotomies have on birth outcomes. The systematic review found no increased benefit to mother or baby with the use of an episiotomy. In fact, the review found that in many cases outcomes are far worse after the use of an episiotomy, with the complications far outweighing any potential benefit. With new research showing a decreased benefit and an increased risk with routine episiotomies, the ACOG has issued new guidelines on their use. The new guidelines caution against routine use of episiotomy as the risks had been previously significantly underestimated (ACOG 2006). Regardless of the ACOG guidelines, it is estimated that close to 35 % of vaginal births in the USA continue to involve an episiotomy (Martin et al. 2009).

Cesarean Section

Cesarean section (c-section) is the most common operating room procedure in the USA (Pfuntner et al. 2013), and as such deserves to be discussed at length in order to ascertain its actual medical necessity. By 2012, the incidence of births via c-section was nearly 33 % (Chmell 2012). This percentage represents a doubling over the past two decades (2012). Bailit et al. (2010) studied the effect unlabored c-sections had on neonatal outcomes. After adjusting for maternal characteristics, the research showed that babies born via unlabored c-section had an almost fivefold increased risk of ending up on a ventilator.

Babies delivered via c-section are more likely to develop pulmonary complications than those delivered vaginally. Infants born via c-section do not experience the compression of the thoracic cage that would occur during a vaginal delivery. This compression of the thoracic cage that occurs during vaginal birth allows lung fluid to be expressed out of the lungs of the neonate. Without compression of the thoracic cage and subsequent expression of lung fluid, neonates are at an increased risk of pulmonary complications (Faxelius et al. 1983). Additionally, historical research has indicated that specific hormones secreted during labor may play an important role in neonatal lung function. Catecholamines are hormones produced by the adrenal glands. They are typically secreted during times of stress or trauma. The main catecholamines are dopamine, norepinephrine, and epinephrine (adrenaline). Catecholamine levels have been shown to be lower in neonates born via c-section versus those born vaginally (Kobayashi et al. 2014). Catecholamines in general have been shown to improve the ability of lung tissue to absorb fluids. Adrenaline, in particular, initiates absorption of lung fluid (Barker and Olver 2002). Inadequate compression of the thoracic cage, combined with a reduced ability to absorb the lung fluid, places neonates delivered via c-section at an increased risk of respiratory complications.

The ACOG has outlined the most common medical indications for a c-section. In addition to labor arrest and abnormal fetal heart rate, the less medically urgent indications likely to end in a c-section are fetal malpresentation (i.e., breech presentation), fetal macrosomia, excessive maternal weight gain, twin gestation, and herpes simplex virus infection of the mother (Caughey et al. 2014). Historically, if the laboring woman or her fetus presented with any of the above indications, a c-section was thought to be the indicated route of delivery. Recently, the ACOG has issued new guidelines outlining the steps physicians and pregnant women can take in order to reduce or eliminate the need for c-sections in these conditions (2014).

Babies delivered via c-section are also at an increased risk of a depressed immune system and of developing infections. Babies delivered via c-section do not have the opportunity to come in contact with the maternal vaginal microbiota. The gastrointestinal tract of the neonate is sterile or has a very limited amount of microbiota. During vaginal birth, bacteria from the mother colonize the infant's gastrointestinal tract through contact with the vaginal and intestinal wall. This initial colonization allows for the development of a healthy microbiota in the infant, possibly decreasing the infant's chances of developing respiratory infections soon after birth. Infants born via c-section do not have this direct contact with the mother's microbiota. This lack of first exposure to healthy microbiota can lead to a slowed development of the immune system and an increased risk of developing infections soon after birth (Salminen et al. 2004).

With regard to the health of the mother, complications from a c-section can range from blood clots, longer recovery time, and excessive bleeding to postsurgical infection. Postsurgical infection after c-sections accounts for higher rates of hospital readmission when compared with vaginal birth, 1.41 % versus 0.33 %, respectively (Ophir et al. 2008). Post c-section infection rates are three times higher than those for vaginal delivery (Caughey et al. 2014). Postsurgical infections are a significant cause of maternal morbidity, leading to complications such as pyelonephritis, mastitis, and thrombophlebitis (Berg et al. 2010). Limiting the number of c-sections to only those explicitly medically necessary can significantly reduce the rate of postsurgical infection rates and associated complications.

Giving women full and recent information about all the different risks associated with interventions before and during labor is essential. However, during labor, it can be difficult for a woman to speak up regarding her wishes toward medical interventions. It is important for discussions to take place prior to labor, with both the physician and the patient collaborating on the birth plan.

Shared Decision-Making

In addition to the increased use of medical intervention discussed previously, the medicalization of childbirth has led to a decrease in shared decision-making opportunities for the mother. Shared decision-making is "a collaborative process that allows patients and their providers to make health care decisions together taking into account the best scientific evidence available, as well as the patient's values and preferences" (Informed Medical Decisions Foundation 2015). Shared decision-making is built on the construct that all participants are experts. Medical care outside of the shared decision-making model places the physician as the source of expertise. The patient is seen as a consumer of medical care, expected to listen to "the expert" physician and follow the treatment guidelines set forth by the medical staff. Identifying the patient in a role of expert is a cornerstone of shared decision-making.

Recognizing the important role the patient plays in decision-making is especially important during labor and delivery. Labor is a highly personal and emotional event. Allowing women to take part in decision-making, before and during labor, can lead to decreased anxiety, decreased conflict between patient and provider, and overall increased positive feelings of the childbirth experience (Say et al. 2011). Henderson and Redshaw (2013) studied the effects the emotional well-being of the mother during labor may have on positive birth outcomes. Data analysis showed that women who were provided with timely information about the process of labor and who were involved in decision-making were more likely to rate their postpartum health more positively. Mothers who not only actively participate in medical decisions during their labor but also take accountability for their own birth process feel more confident and develop a greater sense of maternal identity (Howarth et al. 2011). This research reflects the overall positive impact that shared decision-making can have on medical outcomes.

Addressing the emotional and educational needs of the laboring mother can provide an environment that allows the mother to feel empowered and trust her body's natural birthing process. Attending to the emotional well-being of the mother has also been shown to reduce the duration of labor and the need for unnecessary medical intervention, and increases success with breast-feeding (Hodnett et al. 2012). Doulas, or labor support women, are trained to provide both educational and emotional support during labor and the immediate postpartum period. Providing a constant, supportive presence and empowering the birthing woman to ask questions have been shown to lead to a more positive birthing process and outcome (Klaus and Klaus 2010).

Doula Outcomes

The labor support woman, as the paraprofessional with training in labor support, has recently emerged within the medical research literature as an intervention aimed at addressing negative birth outcomes for women. Medical studies, such as the randomized control trials of Kennell and Klaus, have been monumental in asserting that labor support, such as the support offered by a doula, improved maternal and infant outcomes such as shorter length of labor, greater number of natural vaginal deliveries, lower epidural rates, lower rates of c-sections, increased rates of breast-feeding, and lower rates of maternal fever and extended infant stays in the hospital. The medical research on doulas highlighted these outcomes but offered little substantive explanations or examinations of the role that doulas played in childbirth.

The "discovery" of the doula within the medical domain is largely attributed to the work of Kennell and Klaus in the 1970s. Initially interested in mother–infant bonding, researchers noticed that outcomes differed in births with observers. This led to research questions exploring the role of labor attendants and birth outcomes. Subsequently, an interest in ameliorating high rates of negative maternal and infant outcomes led to the doula being studied as a medical "intervention." Surprisingly to the medical establishment, Kennel and Klaus found that doulas impacted both maternal and infant outcomes in birth. Subsequently, over the past two decades, 12 randomized control trials have assessed the impact of doulas upon birth outcomes, reinforcing the clinical value of continuous emotional and physical support during childbirth (Scott et al. 1999). The research has shown the following results of doulas upon a woman's labor: an increase in positive feelings about labor (Hofmeyer et al. 1991), a decrease in analgesic medication (Kennell et al. 1991; Hodnett et al. 2012; Sosa et al. 1980), a decrease in medical intervention (such as c-sections), and a decrease in maternal tension and time in labor (Kennell et al. 1991; Sosa et al. 1980).

The research also demonstrated that when women were attended by a doula, a person specifically addressing the woman's emotional needs, outcomes for both mother and baby were improved (Hofmeyer et al. 1991; Kennell et al. 1991; Hodnett et al. 2012; Sosa et al. 1980). The doula as an intervention, in all 12 studies, was a "trained laywoman, professional midwife, or student midwife, who provided continuous emotional, informational, and non-medical physical support to laboring women" (Scott et al. 1999). Studies where women were not trained have also shown similar results. For example, in examining the use of female companionship in labor, Madi et al. (1999) concluded that companionship in labor was more culturally appropriate for women, making the stressful effects of the hospital less evident. Within the experimental group, the presence of a companion prevented the medical staff from using early interventions, while in the control group, the staff could focus more "attention on the control group, resulting in increased intervention" (Madi et al. 1999, p.7).

A meta-analysis of the research on doulas found that the presence of a supportive person who had no prior social relationship (such as a family member or friend) with the laboring mother significantly reduced the duration of labor, need for pain relief medication, and use of forceps or vacuum, and the newborn was more likely to have a 5-minute Apgar score of greater than seven (Hodnett et al. 2012). Another meta-analysis found that "continuous social support during labor and delivery had a significantly greater beneficial impact on childbirth outcomes than intermittent support" (Scott et al. 1999, p.1259). This study further described that intermittent support, such as requiring labor and delivery nurses to care for an increasing numbers of patients, was not associated with any improved outcomes (Scott et al. 1999).

While nurses are the primary caregivers during labor in a hospital, at present, the "demand on labor and delivery nurses is so great they can spend less than 10 % of their time providing supportive services" (Kennell 2004, p. 1489). Physicians and nurses are in greatest contact with laboring women mostly during late labor and the pushing stage of childbirth, often leaving women in early labor alone without support (Scott et al. 1999). Medical specialization and technical expertise, "combined with the financial drive toward personnel cutbacks in favor of technology," have contributed to reduced time for patient contact and limited emphasis on the benefit of social support, ultimately "reducing the quality of care during childbirth" (Scott et al. 1999, p. 1260).

There are long-term results of the use of a doula in childbirth, including an enhancement in maternal self-confidence and self-esteem (Simkin 1992). We see the indications of the potential for such long-term outcomes where researchers have looked at maternal feelings postpartum. For example, Lefcourt (1984) argues that in the presence of a labor companion, women felt empowered and more in control of their labor because they knew there was a continuous caregiver that could be called on to help if needed. Other researchers have demonstrated that women birthing with doulas were more likely to feel that they had a good birth experience, that they were not tense, and that they coped very well during labor in comparison with women who were not provided emotional and physical support by a doula (Gordon et al. 1999; Hodnett et al. 2012). Researchers have also suggested that women's impressions of the psychosocial care they received remained quite constant over time, and when these impressions were positive, the women's overall impression of their births became even more positive as time passed (Waldenstrom 2004; Simkin 1991).

The empowerment noted in labor carried over into the postpartum period, where researchers found: enhanced mother–infant bonding (Hofmeyer et al. 1991; Kennell et al. 1991; Sosa et al. 1980), decreased neonatal problems (Kennell et al. 1991; Sosa et al. 1980), increased feelings of acceptance of the baby (Hofmeyer et al. 1991; Sosa et al. 1980), increased cooperation and participation by the mother, and decreased occurrence of postpartum depression (Wolman 1991). Ultimately, Scott et al. (1999) concluded that "given the clear benefits and no known risks associated with doula support, every effort should be made to ensure that all laboring women receive support, not only from those close to them but also from specially trained caregivers" (Scott et al. 1999, p. 3).

Literature regarding labor support women and subsequent birth outcomes was also found within the midwifery literature. This article however referred to a general category of labor support and did not specifically address doulas in the exclusive role of labor support. This is probably due to the role that midwives, and specifically home-birth midwives, assume in offering intensive labor support as part of their philosophy of care. However, in the case of the USA, with 99.28 % of all American women giving birth in a hospital (MacDorman et al. 2012), very few women birth at home with constant midwifery care. Likewise, in the American hospital setting, the labor and delivery nurse is still the primary caregiver with more patient contact than nurse-midwives or obstetricians.

Learning About the Doula's Role and the Relationship Between Women and Doulas

This book stands out because the methods of research we used to explore the role of the doula in childbirth did not follow the same design used in studies looking for causality. Most research on the positive outcomes of using doulas for labor support used randomized control trials and controlled experimental models to demonstrate causality (Gordon et al. 1999; Scott et al. 1999; Zhang et al. 1996; Kennell et al. 1991; Klaus et al. 1986). Medical research findings suggested that the use of a doula positively resulted in better birth outcomes for the women that used them. However, in research that controlled for the women's role in birth and measured only the doula's impact upon the women, positive birth outcomes are "accredited" to the use of an intervention, the doula. This stands in contrast to how doulas actually see their own role, of working with women, and the value they place on the woman's body as being resilient and capable.

The birthing woman, and her relationship to her labor support, received no credit for the resulting positive outcomes, which are the woman's outcomes. Increased rates of breast-feeding, fewer medical interventions, and increased maternal attachment were all outcomes the woman, and specifically her body, accomplished. Yet in medical research, the laboring woman's birth experience and specifically her outcomes are quantified and then those outcomes are accredited to the intervention of another person, the doula. This work takes an alternative perspective: instead of searching for 'what causes better outcomes when a doula is present,' it seeks to know 'what happens when women and their doulas work together.' The only way to understand this relationship is to understand the meaning that women ascribe to the experience of childbirth with a doula—the only way to understand the meaning a person ascribes to an experience is through qualitative research methods.

This book also privileges the voices of women that assert their own critiques of their hospital-based childbirths and appreciation for their labor support women. The ethnographic fieldwork, in-depth interviews, documents, and extensive time in the field resulted in hundreds of pages of data after over almost 2 years of talking to women about childbirth with a doula. These narratives cannot be generalized to suggest every woman that has a doula for labor support will have this exact experience, and the philosophy of doulas that this study reveals will not resonate with every doula. You as the reader can determine what the words of these women reveal about childbirth (as we offer our interpretation) and decide if indeed the critique of the medicalization and alienation of childbirth is convincing; doulas provide a fundamentally different model of care based on love and advocacy, and women are looking for an alternative that values who they are in the birthing process, which is why they choose doulas.

Site

This study combined in-depth ethnographic fieldwork with supplemental post-fieldwork interviews. The study received institutional review board approval and participants signed informed consent forms to be observed and interviewed. All quotes in this text were given with informed consent and participants were given pseudonyms to maintain anonymity. Participants were primarily recruited from a doula-run birth education center located in a medium-sized city. The center offered childbirth education classes, prenatal and postnatal exercise, breast-feeding support, postpartum support groups, parenting support, mother–baby playtime, and referrals to midwives, birth doulas, and postpartum doulas. This was a nonprofit agency with a goal of providing women with more information on childbirth and connecting women to other support networks that would provide professional connections and information on natural childbirth and postpartum-related concerns and encourage and support breastfeeding. Recruitment of all participants was based upon snowballing techniques, subsequent contacts made from previous participants' recommendations (Robson 2002). This method of recruitment often occurred during observation times at the local childbirth organization and through referrals from other participants after interviews concluded.

After the primary ethnographic fieldwork was completed and analyzed, we supplemented with additional recruitment, expanding the interviews to include nurses, partners, and doulas outside the immediate region as a means to validate the original patterns and themes that emerged from the fieldwork. Post-fieldwork interviews were collected via informal networks targeting doulas, nurses, and partners not associated with the hospital or childbirth organization in the region of the medium-sized city.

The primary childbirth organization used for recruitment described its purpose of educating, supporting, and empowering women, new mothers, and their families in making informed decisions throughout childbearing and early parenting. According to their promotion materials, their mission is based upon a philosophy that views birth as a fundamentally normal and natural event, referencing the midwifery model of care, in which women experience birth physically, emotionally, and spiritually. The organization's philosophy also supports the right of women to make informed decisions about their health care. Organization materials describe that the way a woman is treated during her labor and birth has a profound effect upon her view of her baby and herself as a mother and woman. Information materials stated that nothing is more important for the relationship between mother and child than how the woman feels about the process of birth and the first moments with her baby.

We used the term "birthing women" instead of mother to locate birthing women as first and foremost women, before identifying her based upon a relation to another, such as the mother to her child. This does not attempt to reflect that women's identities as mothers are less valid than their identities as women, or an attempt to impose a hierarchy. Instead, it is an attempt to recognize the ability for participants in the study to "self-represent," representing oneself through the expression of one's moral and affective orientation, which can be actualized and effectively represented (Cornell 1998).

We attempted to recruit the most diverse sample possible, looking for nonwhite, unmarried women of lower-socioeconomic status to participate. However, only one participant fit these attributes. Nevertheless, this sample is representative of the clients attending the doula-led organization. Likewise, both the demographics of doulas and mothers in this study generally fit the larger American demographic of doulas, who are predominately white, married, middle-class women (Morton 2002).

Participants

Doula participants in this study (15 in all) were all white women. Most women were married with children, with spousal income. Overall, these doulas generally served a demographic that is similar: white, married, professional, middle- to upper-class women. In the analysis, the homogeneity with which doulas described their work was striking. In discussing their views of what doula work entailed and how they specifically served women, the descriptions by doulas were remarkably similar. In the findings, the apparent consensus of doulas does not represent a generalization to all doulas, merely to the doulas within this community. The articulation of the consensus by doulas, represented in the findings, more closely resembles their homogeneity, and it is posited that more diverse or heterogeneous populations of doulas may offer more diversity in perspectives.

However, there were differences that did emerge among the doula respondents. There were considerable differences when doulas described the limitations in doula work, especially among doulas no longer working with clients. There was also significant divergence in opinion when doulas described certification and training requirements.

Among the participant mothers, there was more heterogeneity in views regarding hospital care, while, overall, the women were consistently positive about all aspects of doula care. The consensus of a positive perspective on doula care represents the small number of respondents and the method of sampling. However, the general research literature does reflect that women report more satisfaction with doula care in comparison with hospital care (Madi et al. 1999; Spiby et al. 1999).

Laura, as founder of the organization, played a substantial role in training doulas and organizing doula services in the area. She does trainings throughout the state since she is certified as a doula trainer, a level of certification requiring further education, training, and commitment to a national-level doula organization. Partially due to her qualifications and partially due to the small number of doulas in the area, in the past, Laura had been involved in some aspects of training for all the doulas recruited in this study. Laura had also participated in a variety of volunteer positions related to doula work, such as working with groups on postpartum mood disorders and midwifery issues in the state.

Sarah had volunteered with the organization in the past as a childbirth educator, but at the time of the study, she worked full time as a paid employee of a local hospital in outreach and community education. She recently stopped taking doula clients due to this full-time employment. Before this, she had worked extensively in childbirth education and teen pregnancy issues in the area. She is white, mid-thirties, has a university degree, is married to a professional, and has children.

Megan worked part time with the organization. In this position, Megan oversaw retail operations and maintained the working office, answering client inquiries and keeping financial records. She also taught childbirth education classes as volunteer and recruited doula clients through the organization. Megan was a resident of the area, yet she began her doula work in another state before returning to the area to practice. Megan is white, late twenties, college educated, not married, and worked part time as a massage therapist.

Jackie had volunteered in the past as a childbirth educator. She considered herself a part-time doula and full-time homeschool mother. She no longer took doula clients due to the lack of financial stability in doula work. She explained that the commitment of time required and additional financial expenses of securing childcare when she was with clients led to her postponing taking on current clients. Ultimately, the amount she earned was not enough to provide incentive to continue. She is white, late thirties, college educated, and married with children.

Jennifer owns her own business as a massage therapist, working as a birth doula only part time. Most of her doula clients were also her massage therapy clients, and she saw her training as a massage therapist as a benefit to her doula clients. According to Jennifer, she focused a lot of her support work in birth around massage. She is white, early thirties, not married, no children, and has completed some postsecondary education.

Kristy described herself as a full-time doula. Her interest in doula work reflected a future aspiration in midwifery. She had been a doula for several years and was currently studying toward certification as a lay midwife. She is white, late thirties, married with children, and has a college degree.

Debora identified herself as a full-time mother and only most recently stopped taking doula clients. She volunteered teaching childbirth education and was a participant of a doula study group. She identified her intention to return when her children were older. She is white, early forties, married with children, and has a college degree.

Heather worked full time for a community health agency and is a part-time doula. She trained with Laura, attending a doula workshop that was observed in the study. Her interest in doula work was a reflection of her interest in women's health, breast-feeding, and postpartum depression support. She is white, mid-thirties, married, no children, and has a college degree.

Susan also attended the doula training that was observed in this study. Her work as a doula involved working with low-income women. She is white, late twenties, not married, no children, with some postsecondary education.

Darlene has been working as a doula for 12 years. She works full time as a doula and part time as a fitness instructor. Prior to becoming a doula, she had limited experience working with pregnant women. Darlene worked with a doula during her first pregnancy, which is what sparked her interest in becoming a doula. She is white, mid-thirties, married, and has three children. Darlene has a 4-year college degree in a nonmedical field.

Beth has been a doula for 7 years. She works full time as a doula. Beth had limited experience with pregnant women prior to becoming a doula. She used a doula for both of her pregnancies. Beth is white, married with two children. She completed 1 year of community college.

Jennifer is fairly new to practicing as a doula. She has been working as a doula for just over 1 year. Jennifer began studying the role of doulas after her first, highly medicalized, labor. She is white, married with three children. Jennifer has a high school diploma.

Courtney has been working full time as a doula for 9 years. During her third pregnancy, Courtney was told about a local doula and she began working with her. Her personal work with the doula led her to begin working toward her doula certification. Courtney is white, married with three children. She has a master's degree in a nonmedical field.

Nancy had no experience working with pregnant women prior to becoming a doula 7 years ago. She works full time as a doula. Nancy is also a certified herbalist and works with her clients to incorporate her extensive knowledge into her doula care. She is white, married with two children. She has an associate's degree in a nonmedical field.

Stephanie has been working as a full-time doula for 5 years. She used a doula during all three of her pregnancies. Her personal work with a doula led her to become interested in supporting women. She is white, married with three children. She completed 2 years of a 4-year college degree in a nonmedical field.

Julie has been working as a self-employed doula for 11 years, although she indicates she works "less than part-time" as a doula in order to be more available to her family. Her interest in becoming a doula stemmed from participating in a highly medical birth of a family member. She decided she wanted a different model of care for her own pregnancies. Julie is white, married with two children. She has a master's degree in a medical-related field.

Pseudonymns have been used to maintain anonymity. The description of women participants in this study will not specify characteristics according to pseudonym, to maintain anonymity. While doulas are depicted with more specific attributes and verified the use of their descriptions in the study, the women participants will remain without specific descriptors, such as age or occupation, connected to pseudonyms. Likewise, when relating a woman's birth story, the doula's name has been replaced with "my doula" or "our doula" to again prevent identification of women based on the doula they employed. Birth stories and their descriptions are sensitive and we attempted to remove, or generalize, any characteristics that could identify women participants. The list of pseudonyms for the women participants is as follows: Julie, Linda, Lisa, Allison, Kathryn, Amy, Paige, Paula, Karyn, Susan, Ellie, Madison, Trish, Ann, Addie, Sarah, and Mary.

The women participants (17 in all) represent a fairly homogeneous group. Fifteen of the seventeen participants are white, married, and college educated. Two women are nonwhite. One woman is not married, currently attends vocational classes, and works full time in the service industry. Two women do unpaid work, one as a graduate student and the other as a full-time mother. The remaining 14 work in paid occupations, either full or part time. These occupations include: health care worker, educator, community service worker, journalist, university employee, counselor, and businesswoman.

Data was also collected from birthing women's respective partners (six in all) and labor and delivery nurses (two in all) in order to gain a better understanding of the process of labor and the need for additional support. This data was collected via interviews and informal conversational situations. The data collected was informative but not the primary focus of the study. The pseudonyms of the male partners are as follows: Travis, Joe, Marc, Eric, Keith, and Jesse. The pseudonyms of the nurses are as follows: Allison and Mary.

Data Collection

Ethnographic data was primarily collected by CH (Cheryl Hunter). Data collection included doula training events observations, childbirth education class observations, informal observations, childbirth observations, individual interviews, collection of promotional and informational materials from the organization, and collection of popular media documents. Informal observations included: mother and baby playtimes, drop-in office hours with doulas, prenatal and postnatal yoga, doula meetings, and organization-sponsored events. CH rotated days and times of observations to collect data from all days and times the organization was open. During all these observations CH took comprehensive fieldnotes, capturing dialogue and interactions. CH also collected education and resource materials used by the doulas when interacting with previous or potential clients.

During this time, CH participated in the formulation and implementation stages of the organization's community-based doula project, attending meetings and working with other volunteers in collaboration with a state agency and a nonprofit organization. CH attended two birth workshops, two doula certification trainings, and two national conferences. CH collected materials from each of these events and included them in the analysis.

The focus upon a woman's birth experience, which primarily takes place within the labor process, is one that is difficult to completely reflect back upon as either a doula or a birthing woman, due to the emotional and physical demands of giving birth, requiring independent observational data to be generated during actual childbirth. CH personally attended two childbirths, in total 33 hours, and watched educational birth videos during childbirth education classes. CH recruited nine doulas (these were the primary doulas working in the community) and nine mothers for interviews. All mothers were clients and all had doulas at one or more childbirths. Doulas were interviewed on two separate occasions and mothers once, with follow-up informal conversations on occasion. Interviews lasted on average half-an-hour to an hour per interview.

AH (Abby Hurst) compiled data collected from nurses, partners, and doulas outside of the region. This consisted of seven open-ended questions intended to investigate the attitudes and perceptions of different participants outside the original research area. Questions were focused on interprofessional communication between doulas and other members of the maternity care team (nurses, midwives, physicians). Open-ended questions allowed participants the opportunity to fully express their thoughts. The interviews were recorded, transcribed, and analyzed.

Both CH and AH used an underlying theory of phenomenology to frame the analysis. Data were initially read to establish meaning units, chunks of data that offered information relative to understanding the role of doulas and the experience of having a doula-supported childbirth. The meaning units identified recurring perceptions and experiences of the participants. The meaning units were then reread for emergent concepts, or codes, and then organized according to emergent patterns across the codes. They were also simultaneously analyzed using the interpretive process of reconstructive horizon analysis (Carspecken 2001) to gain insight into the participant's respective experiences. Emergent patterns, or themes, were then compared with the meaning reconstructions to explore potential relationships across the data.

Transformative Birth Experiences

Childbirth with a doula was consistently described in positive ways and with overall high satisfaction in the doula. Since participants self-selected into the study and were willing to spend hours being observed or interviewed, it stands to reason that the data would be overwhelmingly positive. However, the focus of the research was on how doulas and women established relationships and the perceptions of how those positive relationships impacted women; therefore, it is the positive and transformative relationships that were of most interest to the researchers.

Both women and doula participants regarded and described the birth experience as transformative. Doulas often began describing the experience of childbirth beginning with their drive to their client's house. They described their own experience of waking up in the middle of the night, leaving their homes and families, and driving to somewhere where they knew a baby was going to be born: "It's a very special feeling driving in the middle of the night somewhere knowing that I am about to be at this amazing, unpredictable event. Everyone is sleeping but I know a baby is about to be born. It's the miracle of the everyday" (Laura - doula). While doula participants described their own transition into the "birth world" as one that transforms in transit, doulas also referred to the childbirth experience as "transformative for women." Debora described the notion of birth as a "rite of passage for parents" to convey the transformative nature of childbirth:

> Birth is a rite of passage for parents. Literally, because a baby is produced but also because of the emotional changes in becoming a family. The ultimate crossing of a stress where your baby is concerned. That's a part of becoming a parent. Part of being a doula is guiding them through that special experience, holding their hand if that's what they need. Making sure they come out the other side with the experience that they wanted. (Debora, doula)

Debora describes the doula's focus on the *experience* of birth, and the important attention to be paid upon that experience. For doulas, their focus is solely on the woman and her experience of the birth. This is not to say the child, as a result of that process, is not important, but other caregivers fill the role of oversight for the baby. The doula focuses on facilitating an experience the woman herself would like to have. Chapter 3 further articulates in what ways doulas privilege the experiential nature of birth and Chap. 4 explains why.

Each woman participant in the study made reference to the way that birth had an impact upon her life. The following are just a few representative quotes of how women described their birthing experiences with their doula:

> I just wanted to write to thank you for being there during our delivery. Your presence was truly a godsend. This experience was one of the most amazing things I have ever gone through and your support and guidance were like an angel at my side. Justin and I cannot imagine how we would have walked away had we tried this alone. (note to Laura from client)
>
> There was a real calm in those last hours of labor. After labor I had this overwhelming realization that I can do anything I need to. I look at my baby and cry sometimes. My labor and having a doula was a *big* (emphasis added) part of that. My doula helped me not give up on what I wanted, a natural childbirth. It meant the world to me that I did not give up. (Kathryn, mother)
>
> I am just so thankful for my doula. If anyone is ever in doubt as to whether they would like a doula I am always like, "it's just so amazing" and "it can totally change how you feel about the whole process." I just think that every woman should have such comfort and support through what can be a difficult but transformative experience. (Julie, mother)

These examples describe the women's perception that the process of birth was personally transformative and how they included their doulas in their discussions of that transformation. Women however did not attribute the transformation solely to the use of a doula. Women articulated how their doula helped them "think of things in a different way," but attributed the transformative process to their own bodies. Allison explained that while her doula was instrumental in helping her "to be more aware of all the decisions in birth," "I was the one that made those decisions." Similarly, Paula explained that her doula helped her "reconsider some pretty fundamental thoughts" such as "always thinking I would just go in and have this baby." She continued:

> I just figured that all the decisions are made for me. I never thought I would need to make a decision about types of pain relief or where I wanted to labor or if I wanted them to put in the eye stuff. Isn't that funny? I just thought women go in, have a baby and there would be no decisions I would need to make. I remember thinking, "I have to decide these things? Isn't that their job?" And of course, you take a [doula-led] class and that really

changes things. You realize that childbirth is this *huge* (emphasis added) thing and there is so much that goes on that you have control over, well, if you want it. I remember becoming obsessed at one point about vitamin K shots and reading so much about it. And so I went from not knowing anything and just thinking I'll do whatever they think is best to reading and thinking about me needing to make all these decisions. You know it probably would have been a lot easier on me to not have taken [doula-led] classes, I wouldn't know so much, wouldn't have started asking all these questions. Spent more time on work. Of course, I also probably would have ended up with a c-section, given up on breastfeeding, and without any support. That would have been awful. I am just so glad that didn't happen. (Paula, mother)

Likewise, doulas remind women that the experience is one where the woman makes the decisions and the doula is there to help honor those:

As you are constructing your birth plan take time to read about consider all the different decisions you will need to make. This is your birth, not your mothers or friends, or your support teams. It's your decision and your body. (Fieldnotes from childbirth education class)

My job is really to just give you information or help you find answers to your questions, not to make decisions for you. Try to anticipate those decisions ahead of time and decide on what you want before you are in labor. You may have to change but considering these before you are in the throes of labor is better than when you are working through contractions. What kind of labor I had or what my last client had is irrelevant to what you want. (Jackie, doula)

Childbirth with a doula present was consistently described in positive ways. The overwhelming descriptions of birth with a doula as "transformative" and "life-changing" clearly were of interest and needed to be further explored to understand exactly what made this caregiving relationship so significant to women; what made doulas so different? Why other caregivers are not described in similar ways or have similar outcomes? The next chapter takes up this question as it provides an overview of supplemental data collected regarding other caregivers in labor, namely nurses and partners.

Generally speaking, there are three groups of people who provide physical and emotional support to the laboring woman in a hospital setting. The next chapter discusses each of these groups and highlights the roles and limitations of each member of the support team. Nurses are uniquely positioned to provide support during labor as they are present for almost 99 % of all hospital births. However, increased patient loads, documentation responsibilities, and medical interventions limit the amount of physical and emotional support nurses can provide. Partners and close family of the laboring woman typically know her needs better than anyone else, and are able to speak on her behalf. However, role ambiguity and uncertainty can lead to feelings of anxiety and withdrawal from the partner or family member, leaving the laboring woman without a significant source of support. Doulas are specially trained to work with all members of the maternity care team. They are able to provide emotional and physical support to the laboring woman and her partner. Because of the positive effect continuous emotional support can have on the birth experience and outcomes, doulas are now being viewed as an important member of the maternity care team, with valuable skills to offer.

CHAPTER 2

Nurses, Families, and Doulas: An Overview of Different Roles in Childbirth

Generally speaking, there are three groups of people who provide support to the laboring woman during labor and delivery: nurses, partners, and family. These groups are able to provide emotional and physical support, each in a unique way. Nurses are the primary providers of medical support. They ensure the labor is progressing and both mother and baby are enduring labor without signs of emergent physical trauma. As the nurses are tending to the medical needs of the patient, family and partners are able to provide comfort and emotional care to the woman. They are able to offer comfort measures to meet the woman's emotional needs.

NURSING SUPPORT

Historically, when women labored within the home, labor support women provided comfort and support, allowing for the natural progression of birth. As the process of labor and delivery became more medicalized and moved into the hospital, the role of providing labor support was taken on by obstetric nurses (Kayne et al. 2001). Despite being widely recognized as a key component of a healthy and emotionally satisfying labor, the act of providing continuous labor support to laboring women has become almost nonexistent in modern-day obstetric nursing (Papagni and Buckner 2006). Traditional labor support can include teaching and providing relaxation techniques, giving emotional support and physical comfort, and advocating on behalf of the laboring woman. These roles had historically been provided by labor support women as, until the mid-twentieth century, most births took place in the home, with little medical intervention. Family, friends, and women who had given birth previously were the primary providers of support and care. Labor was allowed to progress naturally, with the woman receiving continuous labor support from a close network of other women (Klaus and Klaus 2010).

As pregnancy, labor, and birth became more medicalized, and more births began to take place within a hospital, the responsibility of providing support fell upon the obstetric nurse. As obstetric nurses are present for almost 99 % of hospital births, they have a unique opportunity to be the primary providers of comfort and support during hospital-based births (Adams and Bianchi 2008).

Medicalization of childbirth includes a variety of medical intrusions, including infusion of synthetic oxytocin to increase the speed of labor, electronic fetal monitoring, and administration of epidurals to block the pain of labor (Johanson et al. 2002). This increase in medical interventions during labor has led to nurses becoming a vital component of the medical team. Physicians are rarely present for the entirety of labor, often only showing up toward the end of labor in order to "catch" the baby. The lack of physician presence necessitates the need for nurses to be present in order to initiate and monitor the medical interventions.

Typically, the physician is present for only a small amount of time. Nurses, however, provide more of a constant presence. As illustrated in the following quotes, not only can mothers find nurses' presence to be more helpful and comforting than the presence of the physician, but nurses also want to be a significant source of comfort to their patients:

> The doctor came in at a few points, but the nurses were more of a comfort/help than he was. (Ellie, mother)
>
> We are all on the same team and have the same end goal in mind...why not work together and have a happy, hearty little family? (Allison, nurse)

Allison (nurse) and Ellie (mother) both focus on how well nurses and laboring women can work together for an optimal birthing experience. Ellie emphasized the importance of having nurses available to her as a more constant medical presence. So while the physician was present at certain points, it really was the nurse who played the larger role of providing medical support. Allison understands her role as the nurse is to provide appropriate care to her patients, and sees the value in working with the entire team of patient, family, and medical staff to facilitate the successful delivery of the baby. Allison underscored how working together toward the same goal of a healthy delivery brings about feelings of comfort in the laboring women.

Even though both women and nurses saw the nurse's role as providing comfort and a sense of teamwork during labor and delivery, the reality of nursing requirements may not offer that comfort or sense of teamwork. Labor support, as defined above, has been reported to only consume about 6 % of a nurse's typical shift. The remainder of the shift is devoted to documentation, medical interventions, and beginning-/end-of-shift responsibilities (Gagnon and Waghorn 1996). An increase in job responsibilities and requirements has been found to be the primary reason nurses are unable to provide continuous labor support to their patients. Lack of training in labor support techniques and personal assumptions regarding on whom responsibility toward labor support falls upon are the other main causes of limited labor support by obstetric nurses.

Obstetric nurses are typically responsible for caring for more than one laboring patient. With each patient, there is extensive documentation that must be completed, as well as monitoring of vital signs and labor progression. The transition to electronic health records (EHRs) has added to the time needed for documentation, with nurses reporting almost 35 % of a 12-hour shift being spent on documentation. Time spent completing required documentation is often listed as a primary frustration of nurses as it significantly diminishes the time nurses are able to spend in direct patient care (Hendrich et al. 2008). Transitioning to EHRs can also increase the cognitive workload of nurses. A 2015 study to assess the effect the transition to EHRs had on nursing care found that the increase in cognitive functioning required as nurses learn new documentation processes could have a detrimental effect on patient care and safety (Colligan et al. 2015). The results of this study showed an increase in cognitive workload for nurses during the initial phase of transition to EHRs. The cognitive workload varied individually, depending on each nurse's computer usage skills prior to implementation. However, even nurses who reported a high level of confidence in their computer skills experienced an initial increase in cognitive workload. This increase during the initial transition period can negatively affect patient care as nurses are required to spend more time "learning the new system," which equates to less time for direct, hands-on patient care.

Mary voiced her frustrations at having to utilize the "improved patient care system" of electronic medical charting:

> I've been around long enough to have experience with pen and paper charting and electronic charting. I'm pretty savvy on the computer, but still find most of the electronic charting to be tedious. Mostly because I'm double-documenting everything. Or at least that's what it feels like. (Mary, nurse)

Mary's frustrations align with what the research shows with regard to electronic charting and patient care. Many nurses report that the introduction of newer technology can significantly disrupt the ability to provide direct patient care. Newer medical technology and electronic charting can double the workload of nurses. The workload of labor and delivery nurses is already heavily aligned with nonsupportive measures such as taking care of more than one patient and limited autonomy in deciding which medical interventions to utilize or not. Nurses may want to provide actual physical and emotional support to their patients, but the time nurses have to devote to providing this kind of support is reduced with each new intervention or policy introduced.

Allison discussed her experiences working with both a hospital with the baby-friendly designation and one without. Within the baby-friendly hospital, there is an underlying assumption that mothers have more options for nonmedicalized births. Many nurses appreciate this approach as it allows them the opportunity to provide more physical and emotional support that they would prefer. Baby-friendly hospitals grew out of the joint initiative by the World Health Organization (WHO) and the United Nations Children's Fund (UNICEF) to promote and support early initiative of breast-feeding. The baby-friendly initiative focuses on encouraging and promoting skills and behaviors that allow for early initiation of breast-feeding. Some of the practices that encourage early initiation of breast-feeding, such as rooming in with the mother, have been shown to increase mother–baby bonding as well (The Baby-Friendly Hospital Initiative 2015). This encouragement and promotion of skills also extends to nursing and labor support staff as they spend more hands-on time with the new mother, teaching her the skills and techniques to successfully breast-feed. The increased hands-on time with nurses allows the mother to ask questions and feel more comfortable with breast-feeding prior to discharge home (Martens 2000). It is important to note that hospitals that do not have the baby-friendly designation are not unfriendly to babies so to speak, but the staff does not routinely encourage breast-feeding, nor does the hospital have specific policies in place designed to encourage optimal labor and delivery and early bonding.

Allison described her experience working in a hospital that was not "baby friendly" and how her roles and responsibilities were in direct contrast to those in a "baby-friendly" hospital:

> Most of my experience was at a hospital that wasn't very baby friendly...the doctors weren't open to birth plans and liked their 'assembly line' to run smoothly. Once I switched to a baby friendly facility...I now have the chance to focus on my patients and not feel like I am abandoning them or not supporting them. (Allison, nurse)

Allison highlights the importance of encouraging baby-friendly policies for not only the family but also for the support staff. Baby-friendly hospital policies encourage mother–baby bonding through initiatives that encourage breast-feeding and other optimal feeding habits. Baby-friendly hospital policies allow nurses to deliver more patient-centered care.

Sleutel et al. (2007) collected data from 416 labor and delivery nurses in order to identify issues that enhance or inhibit nurses' ability to provide labor support to their patients. Nurses were asked to identify and describe techniques and processes they utilize to enhance the laboring experience for the mother. Nurses also provided narratives and topics they felt prevented them from being able to provide optimal care to their patients. The overuse of medical intervention was the primary theme that emerged from this study. Nurses described how the increasing reliance on technology by the physician and other nurses significantly inhibited their ability to provide optimal support. As an example, Susan tells of her experiences giving births: first, with a midwife in a setting that involved very little medical intervention, and second, with a nurse in a highly medicalized environment:

> My first baby was born in a military hospital. They assigned me a mid-wife. This was new to me. I was expecting a nurse and a doctor. As it turns out, I ended up having a wonderful birthing experience! I didn't use more than laughing gas to get me through. My baby was born and we were both clear-headed. I could truly appreciate the moment. For my second baby, I was in a civilian hospital. No mid-wife. I felt a lot of things pushed on me, or at least I wasn't given much choice. I couldn't walk around. I really didn't have much support until my husband arrived. I really missed the previous experience. (Susan, mother)

Not only did Susan feel she had limited support during her "civilian hospital" birth, but she also felt powerless against making decisions regarding her own labor and delivery. With no support system available to her, Susan relates how the process of her second birth was less of a wonderful birthing experience and more of a forced medical event with increased medical interventions.

Mechanizing birth through the overuse of monitoring and labor induction medications can limit the time a nurse is able to provide continuous labor support to the patient as the nurse is now responsible for watching the monitors for changes in heart rate, contractions, and blood pressure, among other things. Responsibility of providing labor support now falls on the partner and family as nurses are occupied with nonlabor support responsibilities, and those responsibilities take them further away from their patients.

Ellie described her experience with what seemed like a constantly changing support staff:

> During the course of my labor, I went through three different shift changes. When their 8-hour shift was over, the next guy stepped in. Actually it was kind of funny. There was a shift change while they were rolling me into my delivery room. I looked up and said, 'Who are you?' (Ellie, mother)

Ellie's experience highlights the concept that many health care institutions are focused on the clock, rather than on the continuity of patient care. The concept of following a set schedule for both staffing and progression of labor does not match up with the construct of providing continuous support to the laboring woman and allowing labor to progress naturally. As Ellie suggested, it is important to provide the laboring woman with continuous support of those who are familiar with the birth plan or the needs of the woman.

Support staff, consisting primarily of nurses, is constantly being pulled in multiple directions. Caring for multiple patients, documenting all required items for each patient, and the responsibilities associated with shift changes make it difficult for nurses to provide the hands-on support that both nurses and patients would prefer.

Partner and Family Support

In this section, the terms "male partner" and "partner" are used interchangeably. This is meant to be inclusive of both male and female partners of women in childbirth. The use of the word "partner" provides some common language to the role of the person who was the primary support person during the pregnancy and will be assumed to be coparenting after delivery.

Prior to the 1960s, the male partner or "dad-to-be" was expected to stay in the waiting room, completely removed from all clinical aspects of labor. As his wife progressed through labor, receiving support from the nurses or doctor, the male partner waited anxiously for a nurse to inform him when his baby was born. Only after the delivery process was completed was the dad allowed to visit his newborn child and check on his wife. This tradition of women laboring without their male partners' presence continued until the 1960s. Gender roles started to shift, and men wanted to feel more included in the labor process. Many birthing education classes and techniques began to recognize the positive effect a supportive partner can have on birth outcomes. The Lamaze method, developed in 1951 by French obstetrician Fernand Lamaze, encouraged significant emotional support and involvement from the male partner (Walker et al. 2009). Emotional support by the male partner allows him to be an active participant in the laboring process and can significantly enhance the birth experience for both the mother and him.

Travis talked about his first birth experience and how important it was for him to be present for the birth of his baby:

> It turns out I was having an attack of kidney stones right after my wife started labor. We discussed it and decided it would be better for both of us, emotionally, if the doctor gave her something to stop or slow down her labor, until my kidney stones passed. After about 10 hours I passed my stones and we were able to resume her labor. I'm so grateful I was able to be there for her labor. (Travis, father)

Travis highlighted how important it was, not just to his wife but to himself as well, to be present at the birth. His wife and he could have decided that he would not be present at the labor, but he understood that the birth of his first child was not an experience he wanted to miss. Travis, his wife, and the medical team recognized that labor is an emotional experience. This experience goes beyond simply birthing the baby quickly, but rather living through the process and emotions of delivering a baby. Travis's experience demonstrates the importance of both parents being present during labor.

As more research became available highlighting the importance of family support and presence during labor, the concept of Family-Centered Maternity Care was introduced in the early 1960s. Similar to the Lamaze method, Family-Centered Maternity Care was developed in response to the highly medical, almost dehumanizing way maternity care was being practiced. The overarching goal of Family-Centered Maternity Care is to humanize and personalize maternity care. The focus of this model is less on medical interventions and more on the emotional and psychological needs of the mother and her support system. Recognizing the importance of family and support systems during labor and delivery, this model respects all members of the maternity care team and encourages the involvement of all members, including the family system (Phillips 2003).

It is now seen as a common practice for the male partner to be present in the birthing room. As recently as 1975, however, many hospitals had policies in place to restrict the participation of the male partner. In 1974, Evelyn and Bruce Fitzgerald completed Lamaze birthing classes to prepare for their upcoming delivery. A large component of the Lamaze method includes significant participation of the male partner during labor and delivery. Unfortunately, the hospital (Porter Memorial) maintained a policy prohibiting the presence of anyone in the delivery room other than essential medical staff. This policy kept male partners out of the labor and delivery room, preventing them from being able to support their partner. The Fitzgeralds sued the hospital, claiming the hospital policy violated their First, Fourth, Ninth, and Fourteenth amendments. Eventually, the courts dismissed the case, claiming the hospital had the legal right to prohibit the male partner from being in the delivery room (*Fitzgerald* v. *Porter Memorial* 1975). This ruling highlighted the belief that a *medical institution* has the authority to limit the experience of a *woman* during labor. This policy diminishes the emotional aspect of labor. Instead of viewing labor as an emotional family event, it perpetuated the concept that birth is a medical event that needs to be managed by medical personnel.

Today it would be almost unthinkable for a hospital to have a policy in place that would prevent a spouse or partner from being present during the birth of his (or her) child. Male partner are now seeking to play an active role in this process. They have a desire to support their partner and also want a greater understanding of the labor process. Attending antenatal (prenatal) classes has been shown to be an effective way for male partners to gain a better understanding of labor and the possible role they can play.

Joe talked about his initial hesitation toward antenatal classes and the value he eventually gained from them:

> I was originally against attending prenatal classes (although I would have never told my wife that). The thought of sitting in a group of people talking about my feelings and fears of becoming a father seemed silly to me.

As it turned out, it was actually pretty helpful talking to the other dads and getting a better understanding of what my wife would be going through. It helped me to understand how I could participate in the birth of my baby, rather than just stand there. (Joe, father)

Joe's experience with antenatal classes gave him an understanding of how he would be a *participant* in the labor process, rather than be an *observer* to a medical event. As Joe demonstrated, gaining a deeper understanding of the emotional component associated with labor can improve male partners' perceptions of their role in labor.

Smyth et al. (2015) reviewed current research in order to gain a better understanding of male partners' perceptions and experiences with labor after attending antenatal classes. Their results showed that attending antenatal classes can not only help the male partner better understand what his partner will experience during labor but also make it possible for him to know how he can be an active participant during labor. Being an active participant during labor can mean anything from providing emotional support to the mother to speaking for her when she is unable to speak for herself (Smyth et al. 2015). Women are not always able to speak for themselves during labor. Emotional distractions ranging from stress and frustration to elation can make it difficult for the laboring woman to ask for what she needs. Dealing with pain and being uncomfortable can also limit the ability of the woman to voice her needs. For the partner, actively participating in labor can move beyond providing ice chips and massages to being an advocate for the laboring woman, and speaking for her when she is unable to.

With respect to antenatal classes, it is important to note that some male partners reported a dissonance between what was taught in an antenatal class and the hospital policy and staff behaviors. Antenatal classes often teach male partners what to expect during each stage of labor. It allows for communication between partners about what each partner expects of the other during labor, and allows each participant to learn more about normal labor. What many male partners have reported, however, is that the classes do not teach what their role is in case something goes wrong. Those male partners who have experienced a labor that did not go "according to plan" felt they should have been given more information during the antenatal classes. This conflict between what was taught and what actually occurred was a frequent complaint of male partners, who felt lost and anxious during the delivery. Frustration at the unknown can lead to feelings of anger and guilt, which may affect the way a partner is able to provide support to the laboring woman. Unlike Joe, some male partners, such as Marc, spoke of the frustration with the practical application of what was taught in antenatal classes:

> Our prenatal class taught us that my role as the dad would be really important and valued during labor. As it turns out, my wife needed a c-section, so the doctor and nurses seemed to want me out of the way. I wasn't able to comfort my wife as much as I wanted. The class didn't really cover what would happen in an emergency. (Marc, father)

Marc's perception that he was in the way during his wife's c-section shows how frustration and stress can alter the perception of what is really happening. Marc was feeling as if his presence was superfluous, and as such may have misinterpreted what the doctors and nurses were telling him in terms of him being with his wife during her c-section. His story highlights the importance of providing clear instructions and expectations to the male partner.

The partner is typically the support person who knows the wishes of the mother better than anyone else present. Being able to understand and anticipate the needs of the mother can increase the male partner's feelings of importance during this process. Backstrom and Wahn (2011) interviewed first-time male partners in order to gain a better understanding of their feelings of helpfulness and participation during labor. When the laboring mother was able to communicate with her partner and tell him what to do, the partner reported feeling more encouraged to actively participate. As Eric discusses next, participating in a specific task can help male partners feel part of the delivery team, rather than an observer. Providing the male partner with continuous information and what to expect during each stage of labor helps him to feel involved. Having a specific task (massage, help with repositioning, etc.) can also increase the feelings of importance and value the male partner experiences during labor:

> I felt completely helpless. I wanted to help but wasn't sure if I should be talking to the nurse, watching the monitors…what? Finally, my wife grabbed my hand and said, 'I need you to be in charge of the playlist. That is your job. Only good music.' I gotta tell you, it seems weird to me now, but having her tell me exactly what she needed really helped calm me down. (Eric, father)

The feelings Eric was experiencing—out of control, anxiety—demonstrate that even the partner has emotional needs that need to be attended to in order to have a beneficial birthing experience for both mother and partner.

Eric's experience coincides with Backstrom and Wahn's (2011) research regarding communication with the male partner. Being given a specific task and not having to "guess" makes the male partner feel more valued and important during the entire process.

Many male partners feel they are expected to understand all aspects of labor, including understanding medical procedures, language, and recognizing their partner's needs during the various stages of labor. To many male partners, this expectation can put them in a place of uncertainty and anxiety. Therefore, also important in helping the male partner feel valued during the labor process is allowing him to decide when he needs to "take a step back" and take care of his needs (both emotional and physical). Allowing partners to decide when to be involved and when they need to step back provides them with a sense of control that will strengthen their feelings of being part of the labor team (Backstrom and Wahn 2011). Recognizing the emotional support or guidance the male partner requires, and allowing him the space he needs to attend to his own needs, is imperative to encouraging active participation from him.

Feeling as if his presence was superfluous, Jesse admits to wanting to step away during his wife's labor:

> I don't think I actually wanted to participate in the labor because I felt helpless most of the time…like all I could do was wait for a contraction and then call the doctor. (Jesse, father)

Allowing partners to choose how much they want to participate can make the labor and delivery a smoother, more memorable experience for both mother and partner. Providing guidance to the partner can help him feel less anxious and more involved in the process. However, the laboring woman's need for continuous support is still the primary factor. If the male partner chooses to step away, this leaves the woman lacking in terms of continuous support.

When male partners are provided with correct and relevant information by the medical staff, feelings of inclusion within the process of labor is increased and they are less likely to need to step away from the process (Sapountzi-Krepia et al. 2014). Providing information and actively involving the male partner in the decision-making process allows him to play an important role by providing assistance to the mother. Lack of information or contradictory information from the medical staff has been shown to decrease the male partner's emotional satisfaction with the labor process. This subsequent decrease in emotional satisfaction with the labor can cause the male partner to possibly withdraw from the process, leaving the mother without a primary source of support. When male partners feel the health care professional is trustworthy and inclusive, there is an increase in the male partner's sense of control.

Keith relates how conflicting information from the physicians and nurses increased his anxiety surrounding the delivery:

> The nurse had been telling us my wife was doing fine, despite being in labor for 12 hours. But then suddenly the doctor came in and announced that my wife needed a C-section because it was 'obvious the baby can't be delivered vaginally'. I don't know why it was obvious to him but not to the rest of us, but he gave us this sense of urgency that we had to have the baby NOW! It was a very different feeling than what the nurse was saying. (Keith, father)

The conflicting information that Keith was receiving led him to experience higher levels of anxiety. His anxiety grew from the conflicting information he was receiving from members of the medical team. As Keith's story highlights, there is an assumption that during labor and delivery, everyone is on the same team and therefore contradictory information within the team decreases the partner's feelings of control and satisfaction.

Role Ambiguity

Childbirth has typically been viewed as a female-only experience. The female was the only one experiencing the physical tolls of labor, the partner was merely there as an observer. However, with more male partners choosing to be active participants in this process, there is a paradigm shift occurring around the view of labor being only a female experience. Childbirth is now seen as a shared experience between both the mother and her partner. Many male partners want to be involved in the labor in order to increase the connection with their partner during and after labor. Male partners have reported that sharing the experience of labor with their wife led to a stronger bond between the two of them (Sapountzi-Krepia et al. 2014). Childbirth is a transition for both the mother and the partner. Both are participating in an event that will change their relationship dynamics. No longer will they be simply romantic partners, but parenting partners. Allowing both participants to be involved in this process can ease the transition and strengthen their bond as they move into parenthood together.

Having active participation in labor also improves the sense of satisfaction men have regarding the labor experience as a whole. Male partners who play an active role during labor develop a stronger parental attachment.

Providing support to the laboring woman and playing an active role as part of the care team allow the partner to feel he has an important role in the process. Being involved in the laboring process can be a fulfilling experience to the male partner. While partners want a more active role in labor, there are no clearly defined roles for them to take on. This role ambiguity can lead to increased stress on the partner. Not knowing what is expected of him can make a partner feel powerless and redundant, leading to overall increased stress for both him and the laboring woman (Johnson 2002).

Effective communication between care providers and patients is important as current birthing practices link both the historical emotion-based support during labor and the hospital-based medical model of childbirth. With the combination of emotional care providers (doulas, family) and medical care providers (obstetricians, labor and delivery [L&D] nurses, and midwives), it is important that all members of the labor team are able to communicate effectively and efficiently. When working within a team consisting of multiple care providers, role ambiguity can occur, leading to miscommunication and ineffective care. Role ambiguity occurs when there is lack of clarity surrounding roles and responsibilities. Within each team, there is the possibility that individual members of the team feel they are responsible for similar tasks. For example, nurses may feel they should be in charge of both the medical management and the comfort care of the patient, whereas the partner also feels he should be in charge of the comfort care aspect. Lack of defined roles can also lead to members of the team assuming another team member will be responsible for a task when in fact no one has claimed responsibility for the task. Undefined responsibilities and perceived overlap in responsibilities can lead to poor communication and stress as members of the team may feel their skills and services are not being valued (Smith 2011).

The lack of clearly defined roles and professional boundaries could lead to conflict between the medical staff and support providers, which, in turn, could affect the care of the patient. Doulas have reported conflicts that stem from role overlap between other care providers. Eftekhary et al. (2010) studied the experiences doulas had when working within a hospital setting. While many participants reported positive working relationships, some did report conflict with hospital administrators and regulations as being a key source of conflict. With respect to supportive care providers, hospital administrators not having a clear understanding of the role of the doula can prevent the doula from being allowed to provide care to the patient. An unclear understanding of the role of the doula has also been reported as the primary source of interprofessional conflict between doulas and physicians (Smid et al. 2010). Educating all care providers on the role and scope of practice and ensuring each unique role is understood prior to labor are necessary to avoid conflict and ineffective communication (Amram et al. 2014).

In addition to role ambiguity, perceptions of the value of care can also affect interprofessional collaboration. Munro et al. (2013) evaluated the interprofessional relationships of maternity care providers. The research identified specific barriers to effective interprofessional collaboration. The barriers most often identified by the study participants included the negative perception some physicians and nurses had of doula and midwifery care, confusion about roles and responsibilities, and lack of a formal structure for working within a team. The negative perception that some physicians and nurses held toward supportive care provided by family and doulas led to caustic relationships between these two groups, resulting in family members and doulas having limited participation in the birthing process (Munro et al. 2013). Understanding the roles and responsibilities of each care provider and having a clear vision of what care will be provided can reduce the resistance to allowing partners and doulas participate in the birthing process.

Similar to what Eric discussed earlier, Travis talked about his role and the importance of *someone* providing him with direction and clear instructions regarding his responsibilities:

> At times I wanted to scream, 'what am I supposed to do?' Do I measure her contractions? Get her ice chips? Stand with the doctor? Stay with my wife? I needed someone to give me directions, almost as if I was a child. (Travis, father)

Travis's feeling of being powerless during his wife's labor matches the research regarding both role ambiguity and stress (Johnson 2002). Travis needed someone to give him a task. Having a specific task he could attend to would have decreased his overall feelings of anxiety.

Male partners are able to provide a wide range of support to laboring women. Beyond pacing in the waiting room, waiting for news on the delivery, male partners are now active participants in both pregnancy and labor. Participating in antenatal classes can provide male partners with a sense of camaraderie with other male partners. The communication with other male partners can help ease some of the anxiety they may have regarding the unknowns of labor. It is important that male partners are allowed to participate in this emotional event. However, if a male partner chooses to step away, the birthing woman still needs to be provided with continuous emotional support.

Female Support

Pregnancy and childbirth were once considered an exclusively female domain. Prior to the twentieth century, women who were in labor would rarely give birth in a hospital setting, choosing instead to deliver at home with other women assisting with the labor. Women attended to each other during labor and weeks of postpartum recovery. Women transferred the skills and knowledge they gained during their own labor to aid other female family members in labor. As birth moved from the home to the hospital, many of these traditions and support systems disappeared as the process of birth became medicalized. Having female friends and family present during labor was not allowed within the hospital birthing wards. The continuous support system that women had relied upon for centuries slowly disappeared as they were now expected to give birth among strangers.

During the 1960s and 1970s, the pendulum began to slowly swing away from medicalized, heavily medicated births back toward more natural births. While hospital-based births were still the norm, more women wanted a delivery and birth that minimized the need for medical intervention and instead encouraged their active participation and continuous support from their partner, family, and friends. Research supports the view of having female support during labor as it has been shown to decrease the need for analgesics and c-sections as well as increase the positive feelings the mother had regarding her birthing experience (Madi et al. 1999). The desire among women for continuous support and education during labor has led to a shift in preferences regarding maternity care settings and providers. Home births have increased by 29 % since 2004, with approximately 0.72 % of births taking place at home (MacDorman et al. 2012). While 33 % of the home births were attended by a support person, such as female friends or family, only 5 % were attended by a physician. This is in contrast to hospital-based births, where only 1 % of births had a support person present, while 92 % were attended by a physician (MacDorman et al. 2011).

Reemergence of Emotional Support Providers

Over the past century, childbirth has evolved from an event in which the laboring woman was isolated from her partner and family, forced to give birth among strangers, to a family gathering where everyone is welcome. Immediate and extended family are participating in this once-private event. There is research demonstrating the positive effects of having an extensive support system present during labor on the mother's overall perceptions of labor. As discussed previously, childbirth methods such as the Lamaze method and Family-Centered Medical Care place great emphasis on strong support systems. Hodnett et al. (2012) studied the effects of having close friends and family present at the birth of a child on the mother's feelings of satisfaction. The research showed that the presence of close friends and family during the birth can increase the mother's overall feelings of satisfaction and accomplishment as the family and friends are able to provide continuous physical and emotional support to her. When all members of the support team work together to create a relaxing and supportive environment, the process of labor and delivery is perceived as more of a natural event than a traumatic process.

Madison explained why it was important for her network of support to be present during her labor:

> I knew I wanted both my parents in the room with me. My sister was there too. My mother-in-law stopped by a few times. It was really helpful to have my closest family with me, they were familiar with the type of birth I wanted, and helped me through the difficult contractions. (Madison, mother)

Madison made sure she would have a large support system available to her. Her story illustrates the importance of the mother feeling supported and tended to during labor.

Conversely, having too many voices and conflicting opinions present can lead to tension and distress for the birthing mother. With male partners, mothers, sisters, and friends now present in the delivery room, there is a changing dynamic around who is "in charge" of taking care of the laboring woman. Family members instinctively want to help their loved one avoid pain. When a woman chooses to have a natural birth, it means she will be going forward with limited analgesics and has accepted the potential for pain and discomfort. This approach can be stressful to the family and friends, not familiar with natural childbirth, to see the woman in pain. The friends and family may try to encourage the woman to forego the natural birth and begin utilizing medical analgesics in order to lessen her pain.

Trish related her experience dealing with her mother, who had a different view of what labor should be:

> My mom was very against my natural birth plan. She could not understand why I wanted to actually *experience* my labor and bring my baby into the world in the best possible way. So every time I had a contraction, my mom would 'tsk' me and basically say 'I told you so...you should have had that epidural...' I ended up asking her to leave for a while. (Trish, mother)

Trish's emotional journey into motherhood was further complicated by her mother's perceived judgment and lack of understanding. Having to deal with her mother's negative views on her personal choices had an impact upon Trish. Fortunately, Trish was able to advocate for herself and removed the negative influence of her mother so she could continue with the birth the way she desired.

Many in attendance may not be familiar with the construct of natural birth. Twilight Births and heavy reliance on analgesics are what many women are familiar with. Twilight Birth completely removed the mother from the birthing experience. A combination of morphine (for pain relief) and scopolamine (for amnesia) was used, resulting in childbirth without any memory of the pain or experience. Women often "woke up" hours or days afterward with no recollection of what happened. Twilight Birth became popular after two American journalists reported on its use in Germany. The burgeoning feminist movement rallied behind this concept as a way to minimize the suffering that women are forced to endure during labor. Eventually, the concept of Twilight Birth lost favor as the risks to patients and newborns became more well-known. Patients experienced risks such as hemorrhaging and slowed contractions, and newborn babies were at risk for depressed central nervous system functioning (Camann 2014).

The premise behind Twilight Birth is the construct that all pain is bad, and must be taken away. The concept of Productive Pain, however, views certain types of pain in the exact opposite way. Productive Pain has been embraced by those wanting a natural labor and delivery.

Seeing a loved one deliberately choosing to be in pain may cause feelings of stress, anxiety, and discord in the birthing room. Pain is typically something that is avoided at all cost. Pathologic pain is associated with something "going wrong" with the body, an indication of danger. During childbirth, however, pain is acceptable as it is seen as a necessary part of giving birth. As opposed to being a symptom that something is wrong, pain during childbirth is seen as a sign that the birth is progressing normally.

Both Ann and Addie discuss their personal experiences of labor pain:

> I was really scared about how much it would hurt. Most pain I've ever endured. It was overwhelming. (Ann - mother)
>
> As the labor pain increased, the nurses came in and tried to make me comfortable. I had a lot of pain in my back, so they thought putting me on an exercise ball would lessen the pressure/pain. It didn't. The pains were getting worse after a few hours so my new best friend, the anesthesiologist, came in for the glorious epidural. If that needle hurt going into my spine I had no idea. (Addie, mother)

Addie referring to her anesthesiologist as her "best friend" highlights how much society has built up pain as a negative event to be avoided, rather than a sign of things progressing and healing naturally.

Within the medical model of childbirth, pain is something to be minimized from the very beginning. Epidurals to block pain and sensation from the waist down are offered soon after the woman is admitted to the hospital. Utilization of an epidural consequently limits the ability of the woman to ambulate or easily reposition herself. The epidural becomes the catalyst to the medical model, increasing the likelihood of additional medical intervention. The decision to receive an epidural or not can be difficult as many first-time mothers are uncertain as to exactly how much pain to expect.

Pain is subjective. There really is no reliable way to measure this complex experience. That being said, a woman's personal experience and expectations of pain significantly shape her approaches toward labor pain. Antenatal expectations of pain greatly influence how women plan on alleviating pain. If a woman has a preconceived notion that labor pain will be unbearable, it is more likely she will decide to choose an increased amount of medical analgesic intervention (Lally et al. 2014). Although, regardless of prenatal education, many women remain uncertain as to how much pain to expect (Lally et al. 2014).

When discussing anticipated levels of pain, women had differing views on what they could expect and tolerate. Sarah explained how her previous experience with pregnancy and loss was what prepared her for labor pain:

> I assumed it would be painful, but I know I have a high pain tolerance, especially after multiple miscarriages. I was confident I could handle it. (Sarah, mother)

In addition, some research has demonstrated that antenatal classes, while effective in some ways, fall short of helping women learn, understand, and cope with labor pain (Madden et al. 2013).

As Mary described, the uncertainty and frustration of not knowing how much pain to expect can lead to negative feelings toward birth:

> I thought my hospital birth classes would help me understand what kind of pain I would be experiencing, and give me ways to cope with it. Instead, the class was really all about teaching us the hospital policies about visitors, ordering your 'special meal' after delivery, and what things we should pack in our bags. I left feeling completely overwhelmed by my uncertainty. (Mary, mother)

Mary speaks of the inadequate nature of her antenatal class in terms of preparing her for the pain. The class had the primary focus on more superficial aspects of being a patient within the hospital, rather than being a woman about to give birth.

Pain is perceived differently by different support people. It is important the laboring woman surrounds herself with a support team that shares her values on experiencing productive pain.

Doulas

Historically, nurses were the providers of all aspects of support for laboring women. In addition to emotional support, nurses also became responsible for addressing the medical interventions involved with labor. The medicalization of childbirth has shifted the responsibility of providing emotional and educational support away from nurses. Obstetricians and nurses are now primarily involved in addressing the medical needs of the mother and baby. It remains important, however, to continue to meet the emotional needs of the laboring women. Addressing the emotional and educational needs of the laboring mother can provide an environment that allows the mother to feel empowered and trust her body's natural birthing process. Attending to the emotional well-being of the mother has also been shown to reduce the duration of labor and the need for unnecessary medical intervention, and increases the success with breast-feeding (Hodnett et al. 2012). Doulas are trained to provide both educational and emotional support during labor and the immediate postpartum period. Providing a constant, supportive presence and empowering the woman to ask questions has been shown to lead to a more positive birthing process and outcome (Klaus and Klaus 2010).

Ellie described how she felt powerless to speak up for what *she* wanted during *her* labor:

> I didn't feel like I had the power or experience to insist we try for something less invasive, but the doctor was late getting to the room, and I was already crowning, and things got rushed at that point. (Ellie, mother)

Ellie described that the doctor was the one with the power to make the choices regarding the timetable for her delivery. Having a support person available to her may have shifted the complete power away from the doctor and back toward Ellie and the rest of the team.

The rise in doula support has been linked to women's desire for a more comprehensive emotional and physical support during pregnancy and labor. Regan et al. (2013) studied the factors that influence the development of a birth plan. The researchers found a need for more in-depth education on childbirth choices and a desire to limit or avoid medical interventions during labor were the main reasons women developed a birth plan that included a doula. The study highlighted that women who chose to follow a primarily medical model of childbirth were found to make fewer fully informed choices about their childbirth. Regan et al. (2013) posited that women who are unable to articulate the benefits and risks of medical interventions are unable to fully understand any possible repercussions of making these choices. They concluded that allowing a woman to fully understand her childbirth choices and to have the knowledge and confidence to ask questions can lead to a better, more satisfying pregnancy and labor.

Developing a birth plan can help a woman feel in control of her labor and empowered to advocate for her needs (Anderson and Kilpatrick 2012). Based on the research of Malacrida and Boulton (2013), women who develop a birth plan are also more likely to choose to have a doula attend the birth. A primary reason women chose to use a doula was that they felt a doula would increase their chances of having the type of labor and delivery they (birthing women) desired.

Ellie describes how she felt almost forced to deliver her baby in the way the physician wanted, not the way she wanted:

> The doctor at the first delivery was not accommodating when it came time to deliver. I asked if we could avoid an episiotomy. He sort of brushed off that idea, saying it would be better to have it. His whole demeanor was more business-like in the delivery room than in my office visits with him. Like he was in control, and not me; he was making the important decisions, not me. I didn't appreciate it. (Ellie, mother)

Not having a doula there to advocate for Ellie during her most vulnerable moments led to Ellie feeling as if she needed to follow what the doctor said, and not speak up for herself. Ellie's situation with feeling "brushed off" after a personal request was ignored highlights how doctors can easily take away the power of laboring women. Ellie's doctor took control of her birth by placing *his* timetable and *his* treatment protocols above *her* needs. Without an advocate, Ellie felt helpless. Having an advocate present could have helped Ellie regain control of her labor, by guiding her to use her words and speak up for her own needs.

Why Women Choose to Use a Doula

Pregnancy, labor, and delivery are emotionally charged, complex events. For the uninitiated or first-time parents, childbirth can be emotional and scary. It is nearly impossible to really know what to expect when you are expecting. Deciding to give birth with as little medical intervention as possible seems easy enough until parents enter the hospital. Nurses, doctors, and other hospital support staff are trained within the medical model of childbirth. Once within the hospital, often times, the woman is at the mercy of the hospital staff and its policies. As nurses and doctors are trained within the medical model of childbirth, the desire for a natural childbirth may not be looked upon favorably. As discussed previously, the medical model of childbirth encourages increased amounts of hands-on, invasive medical intervention. Asking for the staff to approach the labor with a less hands-on approach can be challenging.

A large part of what doulas do is colloquially referred to as "protecting the space." This can mean different things to different doulas and expecting couples, but the essence of this phrase is that the doula is there to protect the mother and her partner and allow them to have the best laboring experience possible. It can be difficult to maintain the special, intimate space that mothers and partners desire for a calm, smooth labor. As explained next, a doula can protect that space by making sure the wishes of the mother and her partner are being respected:

> Part of that 'space' thing is almost they feel like they're kind of in this protective situation ... you know, if somebody has to come—even if the doula is just present in the room—if somebody has to come through the door, the doula is standing there *before* you get to mom and dad. They almost feel like they have a gatekeeper. (Darlene, doula)

Protecting the space is an essential role of the doula. The doula is able to remind the team that the mother's needs have to be attended to. The doula can accomplish this simply by being present in the room. Medical staff and family recognize the doula as the advocate for the laboring woman, and therefore understand that there is an added "layer" of protection provided to the woman. Darlene uses the term "gatekeeper" to emphasize the role she plays in gently keeping negative voices and influences away from the mother and her partner. Information will flow through the doula to the mother only if necessary in order to keep the situation as positive for the mother as possible.

There are doulas that work within birthing centers and attend home birth, yet when asked, many participants report spending a large majority of their time with their clients in a hospital-based birth. It is possible to have a natural birth within a hospital, but laboring women and their doulas need to make sure they are prepared with a birth plan detailing the type of birth they desire as well as information on medical interventions.

As discussed previously, the medical model of childbirth places strong emphasis on routine medical interventions and monitoring. Many doulas report a large percentage of their clients choosing to have a hospital-based birth. The clients want the safety a hospital can provide in case of a medical emergency, yet overall desire a natural birth. For example, Darlene states:

> People that are in the hospital definitely see more need for a doula, and so I think that's why you see a little more skewing of the numbers...being in the hospital system just changes the way a birth tends to occur. (Darlene, doula)

Being in a hospital will naturally increase the likelihood of medical intervention. This increased likelihood is based primarily on the ease of access to the medical interventions. A birth center or home birth will not automatically hook the laboring woman on to a fetal monitoring machine or offer an epidural simply because those interventions are not available in those settings.

Within a hospital-based birth, doulas report having to be more vigilant in terms of making sure the mother's wishes are being observed as it is more likely that routine fetal monitoring and various types of analgesics will be offered, thus limiting the ability of the mother to fully participate in the birth. Nancy explains:

> I feel like I have to help the mom remember her requests a little more often…I am a little more aware of what the nurses are doing and if it's really realistic that they need to be doing it. (Nancy, doula)

Nancy's statement ties in with the role of gatekeeper Darlene discussed previously. Within a hospital birth, Nancy speaks of the potential for an increased use of medical intervention. If the goal of the mother is to limit the amount of intervention, having a doula present to act as a gatekeeper can be a source of comfort. The doula can discuss the procedure with the mother, offering no personal opinion, and review both the pros and cons of the procedure. This allows the laboring woman and her partner to make an informed choice regarding how to proceed with the intervention.

Giving the parents space to make a shared decision regarding treatment is part of what doulas do for their hospital-based clients. Darlene explained why an important part of a doula's role is to help the parents "step back" and review their options in an informed way:

> A lot of it is really just kind of giving them that option to step back from the situation and really look at the choices. For example, if a care provider says, "I think we need to do a C-section," I always talk to mom and dad and say, "If they give you time to discuss it, is it an emergency?" If they are giving you 30 minutes to think about it, it's not an emergency. (Darlene, doula)

Supporting the Partner and Family

The partner plays an important role during labor and delivery. He (or she) is often the one the mother looks to for support, reassurance, and assistance. The partner knows the mother's wishes better than anyone else in the room. It is therefore important that the emotional and physical needs of the partner are met as well.

Doulas can allow the partner to take on whatever role he is comfortable performing. The doula can step in to provide emotional support to the mother while the partner takes a break. She can also support the partner by answering his questions, explaining medical procedures, and providing reassurance. Eric highlighted the importance of his doula's presence:

> I needed to take a break. But I couldn't very well tell my wife, who was busy bringing life into the world, that I wanted a nap. Our doula could tell that I was tired. She quietly spoke with my wife, holding her hand the entire time. I could see that my wife was being cared for, so I felt okay asking if I could step away for a few minutes. (Eric, male partner)

Eric spoke to his conflicting needs of both wanting to stay by his wife's side and needing to step away and take an emotional break. His doula was able to support both the needs of the laboring woman and the partner simply by being calm and present.

Allowing friends and family to be present during labor and delivery can add an extra layer of support for the mother. However, when friends and family have differing views on labor than the mother's, it can add stress to the situation. This is another example of how a doula can protect the space of the mother. Julie reiterated that by gently speaking with the family and providing reassurance by answering questions and explaining what is occurring, the mother can continue to feel supported and confident in her delivery:

> Sometimes it's making sure that grandma is comfortable. A lot of times ... she had a different birth experience and now the daughter is wanting a less medical, no epidural, no this, no that ... and the grandmother is getting tense because she sees her daughter in pain. So it's just reminding them, this is normal, this is natural. (Julie, doula)

As Julie suggested, doulas are a valuable support person for the entire family. Far from merely holding the hand of the laboring woman, doulas encourage a positive birthing environment by supporting the entire family.

CONCLUSION

Giving birth is a complex, highly emotional life event requiring a vast array of support for the laboring woman. Nurses are specifically trained to provide both medical support and monitoring, and emotional support.

The rise in job responsibilities and added workload has led to a decrease in the time nurses are available to provide emotional support. Their role has shifted away from being the primary providers of support to being the primary providers of medical care.

Partners now play a large role in providing emotional and physical support during labor. Partners typically know the needs and wants of the laboring woman better than any other member of the maternity care team. It is because of this intimate knowledge that partners are able to be the voice of the laboring woman and advocate her when she is unable to speak for herself. As this chapter has illustrated, however, the emotional needs of the partners need to be taken care of as well. If the partner needs to step back from the situation, it is important that there is still a support person available to provide continuous support to the laboring woman.

Doulas are able to provide a unique type of emotional and physical support that has been identified as being a critical component of a healthy birthing experience (Gilliland 2011). The support a doula provides is continuous. The laboring woman will have an advocate, a gatekeeper, and a friend with her throughout her labor and delivery when the doula is part of the team. Because of the positive effect continuous emotional support can have on the birth experience and outcomes, doulas are now being viewed as an important member of the maternity care team, with valuable skills to offer.

CHAPTER 3

Alienation and a Challenge to Authority in Childbirth

A full-page color newspaper and billboard advertisement for the regional hospital during the course of the research study read:

> Maternity: Our facilities offer mothers comfort and confidence. A dedicated surgical suite and Level II Special Care Nursery are just steps away from your room, and we're equipped to handle any special circumstances that might arise during childbirth.

Is there relevance of this ad to a study on doula care in childbirth and what is the important to understand in relation to marketing of childbirth? The answer is yes because this ad portrays two important elements about birth in the USA: First, women are viewed as the consumers of childbirth as opposed to the producers. Second, that the medical model, and technology specifically, imposes an authority over the domain of childbirth, limiting women's own autonomy to control their own production. This chapter expands on these two arguments and explains how women have become alienated from the birthing process and their bodies devalued as an authority.

Consider the words used in the marketing ad: *comfort, confidence, surgical, special care nursery, equipped,* and *special circumstances.* The words *comfort, surgical,* and *equipped* describe the maternity ward and also reflect a particular view of what happens in the maternity ward—something that requires *confidence, special care,* or *special circumstances.* While the words describe the maternity ward, they also depict a particular view of what happens in childbirth. These words suggest childbirth is surgical, childbirth requires medical equipment, special circumstances often arise, and babies are in danger. This ad markets to the high-risk birth, where surgically removing the baby, the use of special technology, and a neonatal nursery would certainly be needed. However, it states "mothers" not "high-risk mothers" and therefore is targeted to all pregnant women.

This ad reinforces a fear of "what if" something bad happens which plays on the fear that something bad *will* happen. Standard hospital protocols are often meant to prepare for problems that may never arise, which can disrupt a normal labor for healthy pregnant women (Goer and Romano 2012). "Since hospitals specialize in treating acute illness and injury, they are an obvious choice for women who have complications that require medical or surgical intervention or who choose to have high-intervention births. However, when normal, healthy pregnant women give birth in hospitals, their care often gets swept up into this same medical way of doing things" (Dekker 2013, How Many Women Give Birth in Hospitals and Birth Centers Today section, para. 2). Technology and procedures to assist in a high-risk birth then become normalized for all women and the low-risk pregnancy potentially ends in unnecessary, and therefore with potential risk, interventions

Several participating mothers described their own skepticism about current birthing practices and questioned the need for some procedures such as c-sections and epidurals. Below are the perceptions of Julie and Karyn:

> Before I even got pregnant I had read and already knew a lot. I had a class in my masters about health and pregnancy and that opened my eyes about how women here birth very differently than women elsewhere- for the good and the bad. I also have a very, what's the best way to say this, a very healthy dose of skepticism about medicine and doctors, drug companies, you know. How much we *really* (emphasis) know about all these procedures? Do we really need all this? Do they help us or prevent them from getting sued at the hospital? So I knew that a lot of women end up with c-sections or epidurals because they just go along with what the hospital or nurse or doctor assumes. (Julie, mother)
>
> That's also why I don't have an OB for my birth. You know, as they say, 'to a hammer, everything's a nail.' (asked to clarify) Well, OB's are trained in surgery so it becomes normalized, to cut open a woman, just in case. I mean, do c-sections save women and babies? Of course. But do *that many* (emphasis) women need them? I am just skeptical that

that many women need all the procedures and then who really benefits? (Karyn, mother)

Both Julie and Karyn were already aware of the statistics on high rates of epidural use and c-sections and were questioning these interventions for all women, not just themselves personally. Allison, after taking a hospital childbirth education class as well as a doula-led class, explained one difference resided in the medication and intervention focus of the hospital-based class:

> So, I took the [hospital] class and the [doula] class. Yeah its overkill but I can honestly say that [the doula] class actually teaches you about the childbirth process. We learned so much. The [hospital] class spent the majority of time describing all the different options for medication. Hours describing the kinds of medication possible? Will you get Pitocin, why you would get Pitocin, then when can you get an epidural, and on and on.... How hard is it to ask for medication? It is basically assumed you'll want an epidural and any thing they got. So how is that childbirth education? It more like here's the buffet of medication you get to choose from! What I really need to know is how to manage the pain and work through labor, how is pain different in transition and what are these different stages of the process I need to prepare for? But in a four-hour class they saved all the natural pieces to the last 20 minutes when everyone else was exhausted and ready to leave. The women that only take that class, well, it's sad they really only see one side of it. (Allison, mother)

Allison, in taking both the hospital and the doula-led class, noticed a clear contrast in the medical intervention focus of the hospital-based class. Pairing the media example of the marketing ad assuring medical interventions are "at hand" with the stories shared by women who had taken the hospital-based education classes, it becomes arguable that in this context, the marketing was directed toward promotion of medical interventions in childbirth. This emphasis on particular technologies during childbirth, medications in the above example, frame the way hospitals relate to pregnant women.

The language used in the hospital ad demonstrates an underlying assumption that childbirth is dangerous, thus the need for women to be confident that surgical suites and equipment are "just steps away." The medical institution offers confidence for the safety of mothers from the danger of their own bodies, implied within the cryptic language regarding "special circumstances that might arise during childbirth." Those "special circumstances" the hospital is "equipped to handle" while more explicitly referencing rare and extraordinary complications associated with childbirth implies a danger in childbirth. The danger of childbirth can then be mediated through "dedicated" medical technological facilities.

Much research in the fields of anthropology, sociology, and health and education have identified that American women in childbirth have become alienated from the experience of birth because the authority of childbirth has been assigned to an external entity, namely the American medical community.

ALIENATION AND AUTHORITATIVE KNOWLEDGE IN CHILDBIRTH

Because of the medicalization of childbirth, women have been alienated from the only process that is uniquely feminine, and thus estranged from their own bodily experience. The following sections will bring to the forefront how childbirth in American culture has been constructed and experienced, suggesting the medical model of birth creates an authoritative knowledge system in which women's own embodied knowledge lacks legitimacy and validity (Davis-Floyd 1992; Jordan 1997; Kitzinger 1997). The imposition of authority from an external knowledge system is interrogated from the women's point of view to demonstrate how women can be estranged from their own bodily process.

Doulas used language that suggested to women that they should let their bodies lead the process and mothers were reminded to "not fight that process." Doulas believed the body was not something to work against but rather to embrace and let lead. Paige articulated the notion that doulas encourage women to be engaged with their bodily process. This gave Paige pause to consider if she was actually able to own that process she was surrendering to:

> It was so wonderful to have her there with me, her just being there. There is something special about having her there.... But we don't regard it that way when it comes to the birthing process.... Then all of a sudden birth becomes this other person's domain. My doula and I were just talking about how the woman is supposed to surrender herself to the process.... Of course that is right, but that means surrender herself to *her* process, not someone else's or what someone else is supposed to think how her process should go. She gets managed by this other person. It's like being a puppet. It's your body but someone else is pulling the strings. (Paige, mother)

Paige described a difference between "surrendering herself to *her* process" and surrendering herself to a process that she does not own, one that is "managed" by another. She depicted a disconnect between what she understood as a process where she, or her body, was the expert and a process where she gave up her bodily expertise and another person became "expert." Being managed by another, as Paige described, is tantamount to the alienation of women from the process of birth akin to examples in the workforce where economic labor has been examined.

Women, in their labor of childbirth, are the producers of children, they are commodities to the institutions of modern medicine, and they are consumers of their services but they are not considered experts. Women's reproductive work, in the production of children, articulates the notion of production as described in Engels's theory; the "production of human beings themselves, the propagation of the species" (Tong 1989, p. 52). Marx, however, drawing upon Hegel's insights into the power of human labor, did not recognize the fact that women labor to produce children (O'Brian 1995). Women's reproductive bodies have become commodities, objects outside of the self that possess a value, as demonstrated within the procedures of institutional medicine that attach values to the body as an object. And as consumers, women pay the costs of services as they submit to the impositions of a hospital birth that may leave them with little choice and often no voice.

In an overly simple analogy, birthing women have become estranged from their own labor much like Marx describes the alienation of the worker from his product, locating alienation not only within the product but also *within the producing activity* itself. This alienation is described as a loss of spontaneity of action, as an action belonging to another, and as a loss of self (Marx 1983). The laborer is no longer freely active in any but the most primal functions (1983), and in the case of childbirth, women may not be free to act even in the most primal function. Jackie and Heather, both doulas, offer examples of women and their partners and doulas negotiating their own agency and bodily freedom relative to the use of bathtubs and birthing positions:

> There was either a shift change or something but the nurse that had been in regular contact with [the mother] was not around. [The mother] really wanted to get into the tub. She literally screamed, 'I want to get into some water!' but the temporary nurse said she didn't know and we needed to wait to confirm but she then had to go track down the regular nurse. So she left the room and [my husband] and I went into distraction mode. [My

husband] said 'okay, so its going to take a few minutes to get it filled' and I was trying to suggest maybe a shower might also offer relief thinking what if they don't okay the tub for some reason but [the mother] was not going for that at all. So [my husband] and I are in slow motion stalling for time till the nurse gets back. I decided to leave the room to track down the nurse and at the nurse's station the temporary nurse said that we could fill the tub while we were waiting so that's exactly what I did in hopes that we would get the go-ahead. Which about 20 minutes later finally happened once the regular nurse came back and she came into the room and said we could get into the tub. (Jackie, doula)

When the nurse realized that [the baby] was coming faster than they expected the nurse shouts, 'we need to get you turned around onto the bed, we can't catch the baby in this position' and then 'try not to push the doctor isn't here yet.' While I was tempted to say, 'babies can be caught in a lot of different positions' or 'how does a women in labor try not to push if her body is doing everything that is telling her to push?' But I just tried to help [the mother] through the changing of position into the leg stirrups but it gets frustrating in those times. (Heather, doula)

Jackie described the mother waiting to get permission to move into a different laboring position, while Heather's client was told to get into a different position and then try to stop pushing to wait for the doctor. Each of these examples demonstrated laboring women's loss of spontaneity and inability to act freely; the women were told to wait or where to move. The women's free choice was either delayed or removed altogether.

In a similar example, the woman's choice to wait for labor to start naturally was juxtaposed by her care provider with a suggestion of potential risk:

I have to admit [my birth story] wasn't as I had thought it might end up to be. I had hoped for a natural birth where I could labor at home with my husband and [doula] then a quick move to the hospital just before delivery but of course it didn't quite happen that way. It was after my due date so I was getting anxious about being overdue and on my own a little worried about delivering a bigger baby since he was past the due date. So when I went into my next routine visit the doctor notice a drop in the heart rate and wanted further monitoring. After more monitoring everything looked good with no more drops and my fluid looked good and everything. Then the doctor reminded me that I could go home to wait for labor to start naturally or I could induce to start contractions since I was over my due date. I didn't know what to do. Then the doctor said I could wait but there was always the risk of waiting. I knew we were heading into a time when my doctor was rotating out of the hospital rotation so I think he might have been suggesting that, well I don't know. I also knew that being induced possibly meant other things but I didn't want to seem like I was okay with risking my baby so I was hesitant but then he's my doctor so I told him to go ahead and strip my membranes now. Well that was a real shock, the pain was tremendous and all of a sudden my emotions just kicked in because [my husband] wasn't there yet and I was all alone and it really hurt. When [my husband] arrived I felt a mess but the pain had calmed down a bit so we decided to start Pitocin and call [doula] to let her know where we were and that she probably could wait a bit until things picked up more. I was pretty emotional still and I think she could hear that in my voice because she said, 'I can also come now' and when I started crying into the phone she just said, 'I'm on my way.' When she walked in we both felt a real sense of relief. She was so calm and she knew just what to do with talking to me and massaging me and showing [my husband] where to hold me and where to stand. They traded off a bit taking breaks.

By about 4 am I reached my limit with Pitocin and contractions and asked for an epidural. No one questioned me. I think they both saw how long I had been laboring and I was just exhausted. We all just dozed a little until the next time the nurse came in to check and said I was fully dilated and I could start pushing. I wasn't exactly sure because I didn't really know what to do. I kind of thought I would have a feeling of what to do when they told me I could push but then it seemed like everything from there happened so quickly and once I was able to move a bit I think I could get a better feeling. I think I pushed for about 10 minutes and then it was all over and I have my beautiful baby and [doula] was just a wonderful help to us. I was blessed to have her there. (Sarah, mother)

The doctor offered two options, going home or being induced, and then offered a comment about the risk of waiting without any similar comments about the risk of unnecessary interventions when artificially induced. In this case, the suggestion of risk of waiting and letting labor start naturally was internalized by the mother to mean she was putting her baby in danger. She said she didn't want to "seem like I was okay with risking my baby," but she was also "hesitant" because she "knew that being induced possibly meant other things," referencing potential interventions. As a result, the "shock" of having her membranes stripped and the subsequent pain while she was alone without support made her describe her emotional state as "feeling as mess." Did Sarah have a free choice when the doctor asserted she might be putting her baby at risk by waiting? When Sarah stated "he's my doctor," is she handing over the power to make a decision about early induction to the authority of the medical provider even when the provider may not have given her full disclosure of all the risks of early induction? Where did the authority reside to make the decision to induce, in Sarah or in the doctor?

Birth in the American medical context is *external* to the woman. As a woman labors, the progression of labor is monitored externally, beginning with a timing of contractions to a watch and proceeds with attaching a device to the woman's stomach so that contraction waves can be viewed from a monitor and printed out. A watch, paper printout, or data waves on a computer monitor determine that the labor is progressing. Physical signs from the woman, measured in pitch and tones of vocalizations and physical signs of contractions from face and body, are not considered primary indicators. The woman's body and bodily knowledge in labor is surrendered to the *external* objects that measure her labor. These external devices can receive more focused attention from medical staff than the woman herself doing the labor. Therefore, the labor is no longer her process but a process externalized and surrendered to the authority of the machine and subsequently the authority of the medical institution. While the birthing woman places her entire body into the labor, it no longer belongs to her; it belongs to the medical model of labor, "existing externally as something alien" to the woman "with a power of its own" (Marx 1983, p. 37).

The power of the medical model of labor, and the subsequent commodification of women's bodies, can be demonstrated by data on high cesarean rates for American women. A third of American women (32.7 %) have a c-section (Center for Disease Control 2013), over twice the rate the World Health Organization (WHO) recognizes as acceptable cesarean rates, and reflects a large percentage of elective procedures, not medically necessary surgeries. Healthy birthing women electing to undergo a surgical procedure, opting out of the body's natural process of labor and delivery, is one demonstration of the power of the medical model of labor and birth to define labor as not only an external process, one that can be scheduled and that proceeds without bodily interference, but also as a commodity valued in obstetrics.

The process of alienation as a loss of self produces the relation of the "master of labor" to labor (Marx 1983, p. 143). According to Marx, there must be someone to whom labor belongs, to whom labor serves (1983,

p. 142). If a woman's labor does not belong to herself, then to whom does her labor belong? Who is the master of labor? The notion of a "master" of women's labor relates to the notion of an "authority" on women's childbirth experience. Historically, women have been represented as creatures whose ability to think, judge, and know is without authority (Code 1991). This representation yields a political consequence of women regulated to positions upon which they require "expert" knowledge, even when they have reasons to believe that they know as well as, or better than, the experts (1991, p. 181). Birth provides a clear example of women in a position to rely upon "expert" knowledge and relegate their own knowledge when in reality they may be in the best position to speak with authority.

Similarly, the woman and the medical professional are not recognized equally by the institution or by the state for their material production. This is demonstrated by the codification of the medical professional's role in the only officially recognized proof of a child's existence, the birth certificate. Hospitals certify the birth of babies, claiming the medical professional as producer and deliverer of child. In instances when babies are born at home without a licensed health professional (either certified nurse midwife or obstetrician), the parents must then have the state recognize the birth. This requires documenting who "delivered" the baby. In the case of nonmedical home births in some US states, nonmedically certified midwifery is currently illegal. Fathers "deliver" most home-birth babies. Regardless of the location of childbirth, neither the medical institution nor the state recognizes the woman for delivering or producing her child; it is either the medical attendant or the person catching the baby. Ultimately, in the medical system, the obstetrician is named as the person who "delivers" the baby, eclipsing the birthing woman and her own role in delivering her child.

The following birth story was retrieved from a web-based collection of birth stories. This story is used to illustrate not only the medical and technical procedures that the author chose to write about and include as part of her birth story but also how the writer characterized herself during the process. This story was chosen because it represented a more extreme example of women writing specifically about the medical and technological instruments used during in labor. However, the story also represents the reality that medicated birth is very common in the USA (Hikel 2009). According to the Centers for Disease Control and Prevention (CDC), 65 % of women in labor used spinal or epidural labor analgesia (CDC 2013). In a 2002 study in *American Family Physician*, 44 % of laboring women who received epidural analgesia also required synthetic oxytocin augmentation, such as the use of Pitocin, which speeds up the birth process (Walling 2002):

> I always envisioned myself giving birth without using any medication. I felt that if I gave birth without the drugs that it was my rite of passage into true womanhood. However, the birth of my son changed my mind – forever! When I went in to see the nurse practitioner for my checkup and explained to her about some leakage I had been feeling, she told me to go straight to the hospital. After being checked in and taken to the birthing room, the doctor came in and checked me. I was 1 centimeter dilated with no signs of effacement. My bag of waters only had a small tear in it, but he decided to keep me to avoid infection. Strangely enough, if not for the monitor, I wouldn't even have known that I was having contractions. From 10 a.m. to 6 p.m., I remained at 1 centimeter. The doctor decided to start Pitocin in my IV. I was warned that inducing labor can cause the contractions to become very intense, but I defiantly hung on to my rites of passage theory. I was becoming bored. Around 1 a.m., they started me on Cytotec. I had three rounds, and at 7:30 a.m., the doctor checked me at 1 centimeter still! He broke my bag of waters, and I felt instant contractions. Whoa! I never felt such pain in my life. I tried to convince myself that I would hold out and have the baby naturally. I called John and told him to get there fast. I started off with the controlled breathing techniques John and I learned in class, but quickly I realized that I needed more than breath to get me through this one! Out the window went my rites of passage theory! After a few hours I begged the nurse for drugs. My nice, neat bun on the top of my head was now a shook-down mess. I looked like Animal on the Muppet show through my contractions. Then he came – the epidural man! The nurses calmed me down, and he stuck me in the back with the most wonderful solution to my horrific pain. Ahhh! I'm in heaven now! So much for my theory. I love you epidural man! (Birth Stories, http://www.birthstories.com/stories/2643.php?wcat=35)

The writer described how if "it weren't for [technological knowledge]," she would have never "known" she was in labor. Her story also gives a more detailed examination of how the decisions that were made about her body resided solely in the doctor. The writer offered no examples where she had the authority to make a decision. Even in her description of "begging for drugs," the notion that she had to "beg" reflects a sense that she needed permission from another, hence the need to "beg."

This web blog is not used in an attempt to suggest all women have this experience or revere the "epidural man" in this way but is used as a means to articulate how a woman's labor was controlled and managed by the medical professional, from keeping her in the hospital when she was not in labor, to using medication for inducing contractions, to using anesthesia to control the pain. The medical professional in birth, the obstetrician, has a historical legacy of a male-oriented, and subsequently a male-dominated, economic presence in childbirth.

The charge of high death rates for midwife patients would eventually be used to argue for physician-attended births; however, death rates from childbirth were low in the early colonial period. A midwife's diary in Maine reported 4 deaths out of 1,000 births, while the death rate for men aged 15–44 was higher than for women (Wertz 1996), suggesting women of childbearing age were less likely to die than their male counterparts. Women midwives as practitioners could not receive formalized medical training in schools and subsequently their experiential training came to be regarded as suspicious (Bogdan 1978). Doctors feared that women would prefer their own sex, meaning economic disaster, and began campaigning to exclude women from all medical training (Wertz 1996).

This blog writer described the institutional control of her birth, in keeping her in the hospital when she was not in labor, which demonstrates an underlying economic incentive for the institution. Historically, the medical institution solidified economic power in birth by constructing childbirth as a medical condition, maintaining the economic profits that childbirth brings for the institution.

The culmination of this web blog birth experience was described as reverence for the man who solved the mother's problem and forever changed her mind about womanhood. She closed her story of the birth of her son by saying, "I love you epidural man!" The master of women's labor in childbirth, to whom their labor belongs, resides in the epidural man as he embodies the medical and technical model of childbirth.

Authoritative Knowledge in the Context of Childbirth

The development of the medical model of health care and childbirth as the only authoritative knowledge system has devalued alternative systems of knowledge throughout the world (Jordan 1997). Childbirth in the American medical and institutionalized context has perpetuated a gendered inequality as medical relationships work to disempower women by devaluing women's knowledge about their own bodies. This delegitimization of alternative knowledge systems is a social process in which we come to "see the current social order" as the "way things are" (Jordan 1997, p. 56).

Medical research assumes the birthing woman to be a passive agent in the labor process. Simkin lamented how often, in her career as a doula, she has had to watch women ask permission from a caregiver to walk, roll over, or even drink during labor (Simkin 2005, p. 7). The modern medical institution has pathologized and technologized birth in a manner that views the laboring woman as, at best, a compliant patient. Medical systems function to inculcate individual members of a society with the basic tenets of a belief system, that being the technocratic–mechanical model of life (Davis-Floyd 1992, p. 46).

The western, science-venerating culture of medicine reinforces the belief that the birthing woman is secondary to the technology and the mechanics of birth and is dependent upon "expert intervention" (Code 1991, p. 205). Authoritative knowledge in medicalized maternity devalues experiential knowledge, resulting in what Ketler (2000) refers to as an ideology of exclusive motherhood. This exclusivity persists in denying the validity of knowledge gained through other experiences, whether one's own or other woman's maternity experiences, and rendering only knowledge gained from medical expertise as valid (Ketler 2000). One example is the use of external monitoring. According to Morton (2002), nurses often spend much of the time during early labor entering data into a computer system, and while women have contractions, these nurses spend those minutes fixated upon the electronic monitor as opposed to watching the woman. What might watching the woman's body offer? Megan suggests it offers a similar knowledge about the beginning and ending of contractions:

> It so easy to see contractions on women's faces if you pay attention. You can easily notice the woman's shift in focus, taking notice of a physical change in how she holds her body, the new look of intensity building, and then when that intensity begins to fade and she relaxes into where she was before. While you can watch the monitor and notice *technically* (emphasis added) when it starts, what is the purpose when you can just as easily see it by watching the woman? There are these subtle clues if you know what to watch for and then anticipate based on the signs her body gives you that she is beginning another contraction. Then my attention is never diverted away from her. My focus is on her and her body just tells me what we need to know. (Megan, doula)

While the experiential data will not register the baby's heart tones and there may be the need to monitor heart tones, the woman's physical body, according to Megan, is just as effective in monitoring the beginning and end of contractions. As later data will demonstrate, the sustained focus on the woman also offers support to her, which is highly valued by those that used doulas for their birth experience.

The following birth story from a participant in the study reveals how a laboring woman's own experiential knowledge can be devalued. In the following excerpt, Lisa reflected upon how her expectations of birth were based upon accepting the validity of medical knowledge, from expecting to deliver around the due date to not wanting to accept the medical assertion that she was not in labor. In telling this birth story, Lisa demonstrated how she accepted medical knowledge as the only valid knowledge during childbirth:

> My due date was quickly approaching and I was so excited. I was so tired of being pregnant. And of course, was I on time? No. It wasn't until two weeks later my labor started.
>
> I woke up at 3 a.m. with what I thought was my water breaking. I didn't have contractions at first but shortly when they kicked in- I thought "Whoa, okay this is it." [My husband] called our doula and we talked on the phone through a few contractions and she said she would start getting ready and recommended calling her back in an hour. I do remember thinking, "An hour- that is such a long time! Shouldn't we be getting ready for the hospital? Maybe we should just meet her there?" Of course had I known at that point my labor would last for almost 48 hours, I would have gone back to sleep. I remember [my husband] and me rushing around, but not really knowing what we were rushing around for. I did some dishes and he was doing something, I don't remember, maybe folding laundry. We forgot about the time and almost forgot we were in labor. We called our doula back around 5 a.m. She recommended we call our nurse midwife, which we did and she said she could see us in her office. "But shouldn't I be rushing off to the hospital?"
>
> I finally settled into the idea that it wasn't happening as fast as I thought it was, so we went to the office and my nurse midwife told me that my waters hadn't actually broken, it was just my mucus plug, and I was only 2 centimeters dilated and not effaced.
>
> Technically, I was not in labor. *Not* (emphasis added) what I wanted to hear. I was so disappointed! I called our doula and she was so encouraging that she made me feel like I *was* (emphasis added) in labor, just moving nice and slowly. Okay, that's what I wanted to hear and needed to hear. She was saying to me, "you're right. You know what your body is telling you. You are doing just what you need to, listening to your body." And while I might have really wanted her to say, "Okay you'll have this baby by such and such

time," just telling me that I was going to have the baby soon, really kept me from feeling like an idiot. I mean we were literally rushing around the house at 3:30 in the morning and now it was late afternoon and we were back at our house staring at each other like "okay, now what?"

Our doula was really encouraging; I think she knew how disappointed I was. She seemed to say just those things that made me feel so much better. She said something like, "You sound disappointed, disappointment comes when something doesn't happen. This *is* (emphasis added) happening; you are doing exactly what you are supposed to do, eating and getting lots of rest so you are ready for the next stage." Her checking in with me was so very encouraging. She recommended that I try to get some sleep. I slept for a few hours and when I woke up to a flood of water and then it I knew it. We were in labor. (Lisa, mother)

Lisa's "due date" and the nurse midwife's assessment that Lisa was "not in labor" are two examples of how medical knowledge has been validated as the only source of knowledge in birth, rendering it an *exclusive* authority on childbirth. However, Lisa's story demonstrates that these two seemingly valid measures of medical knowledge were negated by Lisa's actual bodily experience. Lisa's body did not give birth on her "due date." Likewise, Lisa's body was in labor, according to Lisa and supported by her doula, even if in medical terms Lisa was not in a later "active stage" of labor. Lisa's first reaction of "Whoa, this is it," was then delegitimized by the nurse midwife's assertion that she was "not in labor." She accepted the medical knowledge as authority, reflecting upon how much she "didn't want to hear" that she was not in labor and her subsequent disappointment. She did not accept her own bodily knowledge as valid until her discussion with her doula that privileged Lisa's knowledge over the nurse midwife's.

Creating a Discourse of Childbirth as Pathological

Nineteenth-century beliefs that childbirth was a natural process, commonly assisted by midwives, began to be challenged by prominent male physicians, namely Benjamin Rush and William Dewees. Both asserted that childbirth is akin to a disease requiring a cure through medical intervention (Bogdan 1978; Caton 1999). Defining childbirth as either natural care or medical cure had implications in the management of deliveries. Depending upon the labor attendant, a woman could expect vastly different care. In natural care management, a woman would be comforted, encouraged, and remedied with teas, while in medical cure management, she would be catheterized, given cathartics, and bled till fainting (Bogdan 1978; Caton 1999).

The traditionally held view that physician-attended childbirth was safer with each emerging technology was erroneous. The use of forceps most likely caused more death or injury than benefit, from scalping the baby or tearing the woman (Wertz 1996). Blanton argues that before bacteriology was understood, forceps took more lives than they saved (1972).

In the 1900s female midwives became targeted as the source of high maternal and infant mortality, which was augmented by the "midwife problem" asserted by male physicians. The "midwife problem," as portrayed in the 1910s and 1920s and embedded with race and class prejudices, described a midwife as a "woman who goes to the scene of the labor in the ordinary dirty clothes that she has been wearing while doing household work, taking her satchel containing a handful of absorbent cotton" (Bulleting of the Lying In Hospital 1913, p. 23). In the American context, a gentlewoman, offered the choice between a lower-class midwife and a doctor of equal social status, would most likely choose the doctor (Wertz 1996).

Historically, the heterogeneity of midwives compounded the eventual demise of the American midwife due to waves of immigration and variation among sections of the population and their care providers (Loudon 1992). For example, in large cities, pockets of new immigrants also employed newly immigrant midwives of the same ethnicity. With a lack of standardization across these disparate groups, the role of medicalized births gained prominence (Loudon 1992). Out of all of these ethnic groups, only the southern black midwife and two midwifery organizations survived, Maternity Center Association of New York City and Frontier Nursing Service of Kentucky (Bourgeault and Fynes 1997).

By the mid-nineteenth century, midwifery was well established as departments in medical schools, yet beginning in the 1920s, there was the emergence of the academic title of professor of obstetrics within schools of medicine (Cutter and Viets 1964, p. 170). Nineteenth-century birth practices helped accustom people to physicians, while in the first two decades of the twentieth century, obstetrician-attended births helped families become accustomed to hospitals (Wertz 1996). This trajectory of midwifery moved from laywomen midwives to a medicalized and institutionalized structure of midwifery, culminating in further medicalization with the emergence of obstetrics.

One newly emerging role of the obstetrician was in judging a woman's psychological health. A woman who felt too much pain in childbirth was judged to have poor health habits and a woman who felt too little pain lacked the civilization of the middle class, the classic example of painless birth being the Indian woman (Wertz 1996, p. 16). The more civilized and urbanized a woman was, the greater the likelihood of pain and therefore the greater need for intervention through drugs and instruments (1996).

The medical diagnosis of "hysteria" in the nineteenth century, primarily diagnosed as gynecologic and/or reproductive disorders, can be seen as a reaction to women's increased participation in the public sphere and their declining fertility (Briggs 2000). The *American Journal of Obstetrics* in the 1880s deployed racial distinctions, underpinning a discourse of white upper-class female frailty juxtaposed to nonwhite lower-class female hardiness and prolific fertility (Briggs 2000). "Ultimately this doubled discourse of women had profound consequences for medicine and science: the frailty and nervousness of one group provided the raison d'être of obstetrics and gynecology, while the insensate hardiness of the other offered the grounds on which they became experimental 'material' that defined its progress" (Briggs 2000, p. 247). Therefore, it can be argued that obstetric and gynecological doctors owe their professional and economic status for the past 200 years to the women in their delivery rooms (Wertz 1996).

By the 1920s physicians initiated legislation to remove midwifery from the obstetrics field (Bogdan 1978). Medical and state officials began legislating reproductive health in the political and legal mandates that removed midwifes from practicing in many states. The categorization of midwives and home-birthing women as "pathologic mothers," demonstrated how discourses of pathology were created for those who challenged dominant ideologies of childbirth (Craven 2005). Not until the natural childbirth movement in the 1960s did certified nurse midwifery gain attention. The lay midwife, women with nonmedical certification, has continued to be marginalized due to the political and legal structures that restrict her work (Mander 2001).

Labeling midwives and subsequently home-birth women as "pathological" in political and legal discourse while simultaneously describing birth as pathological in mainstream discourse provides an interesting paradox. In the first case, women who give birth at home are pathological for subverting mainstream birthing practices, while in the second case, childbirth in general is pathological, requiring medical interventions. Either description renders women and their bodies as diseased and irrational. In another interesting paradox, women at this point, the early- to mid-twentieth century, were arguing for control and authority over their bodies and their ability to make decisions in regard to birthing practices, manifesting in the Twilight Sleep movement. The Twilight Sleep movement is examined in the next section as an example of pathological agency, the limiting of women's agency within a discourse of female pathology.

Pathological Agency

While this section will address the apparent agency of women in asserting and lobbying for power in childbirth decisions, the decisions that women were able to assert were decisions framed by the medical community as acceptable interventions. A woman's agency was still limited within the structure of the medical system, and in the case of Twilight Sleep, the restriction of women to confinement, contributed to maintaining the notion of childbirth as pathological.

Twilight Sleep combined morphine, to reduce pain, with scopolamine, which removed the memory of pain and, with it, bodily inhibitions. Women on scopolamine typically scream and thrash around, yet have no memory of the experience. This was seen as a panacea for pain in childbirth.

Women saw medicalizing childbirth as a way of gaining control over their bodies and the pain of childbirth. Women wanted control over the birth experience and anesthesia was seen as the answer. Womanhood no longer was rooted in the domestic, "natural" environment (Howell-White 1999). Medicalizing childbirth reflected the struggle for release from the "natural" and thus "painful root of the childbearing experience," in which the "natural way of doing things" was losing its appeal for many American women, and the obstetrician "was there to reap the results of a growing anxiety about childbirth" (Howell-White 1999, p. 363).

In the following excerpt, the use of Twilight Sleep in childbirth in 1914 is described by physician Carl Gauss:

> Even with the careful adjustment of the dose, many women became confused and disoriented with Twilight Sleep. Freed of their inhibitions with scopolamine but still in pain, the [women] would scream and thrash about. I found that I could minimize this reaction by eliminating extraneous sensory input. Women are kept in a dark and quiet room, her eyes bandaged with gauze, and her ears stuffed with wads of cotton soaked in oil. To prevent the

women from injuring themselves, they are confined to a padded bed and an attendant or physician kept constantly by their side. During delivery of the child her arms are restrained with leather thongs and I supplement Twilight Sleep with a general anesthesia. (Caton 1999, pp. 134–135)

The biggest objectors to these practices were often general practitioners. They expressed concern over the safety of both woman and child with the extensive use of scopolamine and morphine. Obstetricians used this objection to discredit general practitioners and midwives, who were still delivering large numbers of American babies (Leavitt 1980).

Interestingly, the biggest proponents of Twilight Sleep were middle- and upper-class women. The National Twilight Sleep Association organized by middle-class clubwomen became a movement demanding the right of women to choose how they gave birth, a rally cry of early feminists to assert control over their own birthing experiences (Leavitt 1980). Most recently, many women under the name of feminism have supported the movement toward elective cesareans. The argument and language used for promoting elective cesareans draw upon the notion of women's rights to control their own birth experience, drawing many parallels with the Twilight Sleep arguments of the 1930s and 1940s.

A countermovement in childbirth emerged with the (re)introduction of the notion of natural childbirth to women in Grantly Dick-Read's 1933 book *Natural Childbirth*. The popularity of Dick-Read did not emerge until the reintroduction in 1960 of his work, as *Childbirth Without Fear*. His book argued that childbirth pain was a product of a materialist and atheist culture in which "superstition, civilization and culture" had introduced "fear and anxiety" in the minds of women (Dick-Read 1933, p. 6). "The more cultured the races of the earth have become, so much more positive have they been in pronouncing childbirth to be a painful and dangerous ordeal" (p. 6). He supported the notion that childbirth reinforces the feminine qualities of patience and tenderness, which are important qualities that serve to enhance the marriage (Dick-Read 1960). The Lamaze method of controlled breathing also emerged as a popular childbirth education model.

Dr Ferdinand Lamaze argued that working-class women who believed and obeyed what they were taught were more successful in the Lamaze method (Lamaze 1956). This supposition, along with Dick-Read, ushered in a new concept in birth practices, childbirth education. While women in the late 1950s and 1960s were more active in asserting their expectations in birth, women's agency in childbirth was still tied to the assertion of passivity and compliance to the medical model of childbirth. The growing interest in childbirth education did not occur until the late 1960s with the convergence of the feminist movement, consumer movement, and back-to-nature romanticism social movements giving ideological support to the notion of a "natural" childbirth (Nelson 1982). Initiated and grounded in the interests of middle-class women for more control in the process and more autonomy in decision-making, the idea of preparing for childbirth was still highly removed from most American women until it gained support from the medical community in the mid-1970s.

Medical officials began advocating and even requiring patients to attend childbirth education courses. Physicians found that while prepared clients might disrupt some routines, they were generally more cooperative during labor, fostering a reduction in medication, which increased the measured safety for mother and child (Nelson 1982). Research on childbirth education is mostly confined to formal educational settings such as childbirth education classes, often those delivered at or supported by a medical institution. This extends the medical institutions' potential control not only over the labor process but also how it is represented to women in education classes.

In contrast to this view, doulas assumed that while complications can arise, childbirth in their experiences was primarily uneventful, meaning external medical intervention is unnecessary, and perfectly natural, that is, there is nothing inherently wrong in the bodily process.

The Counterdiscourse on Doulas

Women in this study described the process of birth as personally transformative and included their doulas in their discussions of that transformation. Women however did not attribute the transformation solely to the use of a doula. Women articulated how their doula helped them "think of things in a different way," but attributed the transformative process to their own bodies. Allison explained that while her doula was instrumental in helping her "to be more aware of all the decisions in birth," "I was the one that made those decisions." Similarly, Paula explained that her doula helped her "reconsider some pretty fundamental thoughts" such as "always thinking I would just go in and have this baby." She continued:

> I just figured that all the decisions are made for me. I never thought I would need to make a decision about types of pain relief or where I wanted to labor or if I wanted them to put in the eye stuff. Isn't that funny? I just

thought women go in, have a baby and there would be no decisions I would need to make. I remember thinking, "I have to decide these things? Isn't that their job?" And of course, you take a [doula-led] class and that really changes things. You realize that childbirth is this *huge* (emphasis added) thing and there is so much that goes on that you have control over, well, if you want it. I remember becoming obsessed at one point about vitamin K shots and reading so much about it. And so I went from not knowing anything and just thinking I'll do whatever they think is best to reading and thinking about me needing to make all these decisions. You know it probably would have been a lot easier on me to not have taken [doula-led] classes, I wouldn't know so much, wouldn't have started asking all these questions. Spent more time on work. Of course, I also probably would have ended up with a c-section, given up on breastfeeding, and without any support. That would have been awful. I am just so glad that didn't happen. (Paula, mother)

Paula did not completely attribute her positive birth to a doula or doula-led classes. She subsequently described in her birth story her role in decision-making, attributing the transformative experience to her own body by saying "those were the things I did that really made a difference in my birth."

According to both women and doulas in this study, the woman's body, as opposed to the external measures of her body, was the source of measuring progress and predicting progress. Julie, in telling her birth story, described asserting her own wishes and her doula's support in labor:

So I settled into the room and then after they examined me again, I was ready to get up. The nurse wanted to keep monitoring and I had discussed with both [my husband] and our doula that I did not want to be laying in bed a lot.... I think I was at 4 centimeters and thought I still had a way to go. And moving had been really helpful in early labor so I knew that walking would be helpful.... I remember telling [my husband] that I wanted to get in the shower at this point and so a contraction was beginning and then the nurse said something like, "we need a few more minutes on the monitor." So [My husband] is holding me through my contraction and it seemed like before it had totally ended our doula was asking the nurse how the heart tones looked, and when the nurse said, "they look good," our doula was like, "that's great, she can get in the shower now." Our doula asked the nurse for the portable monitor. [My husband] told me the nurse didn't seem too happy about the extra nuisance, but he said, "You got in the shower and they basically left you alone for awhile." I labored in the shower a long time.... but it was so helpful to be in that shower. The nurses finally made me get out so they could check me again, but by that time I was almost in transition and I remember not wanting to get out at first, so my doula said I could sit on the toilet for a few minutes and then wham, transition, I think I barely made it to bed.... [My husband] told me I was like, "I'm pushing!" then he said someone hurried to check me and then said "you can go ahead and push now." I was already pushing so I didn't hear that.... I can't imagine being stuck in a bed that whole time. Who knows how long I would have been in labor.... If I hadn't been in the shower, I would have gone crazy. (Julie, mother)

Julie's story demonstrates several things. First, she described having knowledge; she "knew that walking would be helpful." Julie depicted decisions made during birth, such as getting in the shower when nurses wanted to keep monitoring her, that impacted her birth. She considered her moving around and her being in the shower as important for her progressing in labor. She also made reference to what *she* wanted to do that seemed contrary to what the nursing staff wanted her to do. She remembered the doula assisting her in getting out of bed by stating "great, she can get in the shower now," reinforcing Julie's own decision-making process.

Second, Julie considered her decisions to have had an impact on her labor. Her comment of "If I hadn't been in the shower" implied that she would not have been happy if she had stayed in bed. She also connected her showering, which was her decision and supported by her husband and doula, to a faster labor. Of course, asking whether or not the shower actually made labor faster is not as important as recognizing that Julie's perception of her labor was affected by asserting her decision to get out of bed.

What is also interesting in Julie's story is that Julie recognized that she was ready to begin pushing before she was officially "told to." Her partner described how someone had to quickly check her and give her permission, even though she was actually already pushing. This exhibits how Julie's bodily knowledge became secondary to the assessment of medical knowledge. Permission to push was not given to Julie until the medical staff had "checked" her, reinforcing the external authority of the medical staff over the bodily feeling of the mother.

Inherent in this notion that women's bodies "drive" the experience is a belief that women's bodies are inherently capable of giving birth and the majority of women do not need interference. Doulas assumed women's bodies were capable of birthing without intervention, aligning with the

WHO suggestion that "generally, between 70 % and 80 % of all pregnant women may be considered as low-risk at the start of labor" (WHO 1996). This is not to assert that doulas assumed women *should* give birth without intervention, but rather they assumed the female body in general did not require intervention. The underlying philosophy of doula care stands in contrast to how the medical institution views the female body, as deficient and in need of intervention from an external authority.

In comparison, the relationship that birthing women participants had with their doulas mirrored the relationship women had with other care professionals, such as nurses, obstetricians, midwifes, or childbirth educators. There was a similar chronology in the relationship, defined by a beginning and ending date, which framed the relationship like other professional relationships. Doulas also provided elements of care in a way that was similar to each other and that care stood in contrast to other professionals. These elements included providing information, listening, touching, and responding to needs. When participating doulas described their interactions with clients, they described meetings where they (doulas) provided information, offered physical and emotional support, offered breast-feeding or infant care support, and postpartum support. It can be conceived that these educational and care services can and are replicated by other care professionals, specifically nurses, midwives, and childbirth educators.

However, the use of doulas, in contrast to other birth professionals, has demonstrated consistent measurable positive birth outcomes. The majority of education and care, described by both women and doula participants, occurred during the birthing event but also extended prior to and after childbirth. While the laboring event has been the focus of medical research, scant studies have examined the doulas educative role pre and post birth. Doulas in this research offered both formal educative interactions (childbirth classes) and informal education interactions (client meetings and birth interactions) that provided conceptual challenges to the medical construction of birth.

These conceptual challenges reside in the fundamentally divergent philosophy of embodied childbirth as intimate labor and teaching of love and advocacy that doulas emulated. Doulas regarded childbirth as an embodied process within an embodied sense of time. This view of regarding childbirth as *embodied* lodges a critique upon medical institutional birth. This critique charges that the woman's body is both the center of the process and an internally measured sense of time, as opposed to centering process and time upon the institution or external measurement.

CHAPTER 4

Birthing with Doulas: The Embodied Birth Experience

It has already been established that doulas play three overarching roles in the childbirth process in terms of education, support, and advocacy. There are a plethora of training books, articles, and online resources that describe the techniques that doulas use when they interact with their clients. These resources attempt to articulate the practical application of the craft of doulas. However, the following chapters are different. These next two chapters endeavor to not only describe what doulas *do* in the *process* of supporting, educating, and advocating for women but, more importantly, understand *why* it is important to the doulas and the women they serve.

When doulas described what they do in practice, they would often say things such as:

> I think what I do is what any woman would do in the same experience, I hold hands, I speak softly, I listen to what she is saying and reinforce she is strong and doing this well. (Kristy, doula)
> There really isn't any amazing bag of tricks. We have techniques that help but it's really more about just being with her. (Debora, doula)
> So, where was I useful, as a doula? I honestly did not feel I did anything remarkable. There were no heroic measures, no advice I provided nor did Sue do anything I suggested. I asked Sue later how I could have been helpful when Joe was there with her, doing everything right: holding her hand, speaking to her in that tone of voice she loves, rubbing her back, and

being strong. She said with me there, he felt empowered to do these things. He followed my lead. Since I remained calm, he knew everything was going well; he provided support when I provided support; he moaned when I moaned. Hearing that, I felt strong, and useful. (PHDOULA 2009)

There may be a misconception outside the doula community, say in hospitals, that all they need to do is to find out what we do then they can do the same thing and 'bang' they solved the problem. But what we do isn't brain science there's no secret doula techniques. We mother the mother and try to hold the space so she has the birth she, and I do mean she, wants. (Heather, doula)

These doulas paint a picture of what they *do* as rather ordinary or commonplace support techniques. However, they also articulate that their practice is not merely a sum of the individual techniques they use.

Doulas articulate a holistic nature of their practice and often refer to this as "holding the space":

And holding the space means impacting the space whether anyone in the room is aware of it or not. Holding the space—*as* love—when a woman is feeling tremendous fear is perhaps the beginning of a shift toward receiving a woman's experience instead of stealing it from her. Our job is to feel our own experience and take it in, all the way, knowing that when we get home, there will be a time to process, to reflect, even to scream and sob if we need to.

Every woman deserves to have the space held for her, regardless of her birth outcome. And every doula has the power to hold and expand that space for her client... without budging. No one can take that power away from a doula. (DTI Admin 2013)

In an attempt to better understand the complexity of the doula's role in childbirth and the various ways doulas describe what they do in their practice, these questions were central: what are the components of physical and emotional support, education, and advocacy; how do they come together to "hold the space"; and what does it mean to the mother to have a doula playing this role?

According to this group of women, mothers and doulas, the doulas' overall practice involved creating an experience that was *embodied* in both the space surrounding the process and the time that elapsed throughout the event. An *embodied* experience is one in which the woman's bodily process is the focus, not to be overshadowed by the impending infant but to be reveled in as equally important to the woman's experience as it is to the outcome of a healthy baby. This *embodied* space and process is one where the woman's physical body is the focus; her bodily process is more than a vehicle to delivering a baby; it is a passage for the woman as well.

In this research the women's descriptions of the specific physical and emotional support techniques, however, paled in comparison with the descriptions of how the techniques, information, and advocacy contributed to an overall experience. The data provide a picture of childbirth with a doula as a holistic and embodied process and the doula's role was to keep that holistic and embodied time and process central in the woman's experience of childbirth.

The Embodied Time Surrounding Birth

This data suggest that doulas hold beliefs about birth that identify the body as central to the experience and frame that experience around the woman's specific bodily process and needs. With their focus on the experience of birth and the central role the body plays, doulas talk about birth and engage in birth in fundamentally different ways than other care providers. The focus on the body rather than on time or mechanical impositions exhibits a model to the mother that her focus should be attuned to her body and her attention directed toward the experience unfolding as opposed to what others may be doing around her, especially in a hospital-birth setting. While no woman or other person can completely plan or direct it, the process does not merely wash over the woman; but rather, she *is* this process (Young 1995). Doulas emulate the belief that women and their bodies *are* the process. The process of childbirth is a passage for the woman and to not attend specifically to that process, with a focus on her capable body as driving it, is to diminish the passage of a woman into motherhood.

Childbirth as viewed from a scientific approach cannot capture the *embodied* birth, the woman *in* birth—only the scientific, static, and inanimate birth as conceptualized by codified moments of birth translated into measurable sequences resulting in a generalized outcome. However, childbirth has not always been viewed as scientific. It was not until the work of French physicians, in developing measurements of the pelvis, and English physicians, in developing the forceps instrument, which gave medicine its first claims to be a science but also brought the application of science to childbirth (Wertz 1996). This has had irrefutable impacts on the nature of childbirth for mothers.

COUNTERING SCIENTIFIC SCRIPTS IN CHILDBIRTH

Blackwell (2001) documented the medical technology used in man-midwifery education in the late eighteenth century in France and Britain in her descriptions of how a "mechanical mother" was created to simulate how to use forceps to remove fetuses. The technology of the time was represented in the mechanical mother, a basket-weave shell that mimicked a pregnant woman's belly from which students could practice delivering wads of cloth from a glass container within the shell. For medical students, it was the "haste of delivery, where nature could be made to submit to the clock, that became the sole measure of success" (Blackwell 2001, p. 92). Blackwell depicted late-eighteenth-century male medical students as taking "center stage" in the delivery of the child. She contrasted this to the newly devised mechanical mother, a passive mannequin in which the child was extracted by another. She argued that with the invention of the mechanical mother, the ideal female body in birth was "compliant and uncomplaining, precisely because this demure and motionless patient is the overinvested primal object of medical education" (Blackwell 2001, p. 90).

In early American medical texts, this notion of compliance and haste also emerged. In discussions of difficult births, haste is encouraged by the practitioner as "all causes of delay are to be removed" (Cutter and Viets 1964, p. 8). In 1724, John Maubray published *The Female Physician,.... The Whole Art of New Improved Midwifery*, asserting that women have finally been taught:

> [t]o lay aside all the childish bashfulness and modesty... to secure their Own and Children's Safety by inviting the physician into their assistance; men being better versed... with greater presence of mind, always found readier to devise something more *new* and to give quicker relief in cases of difficult births, than common midwives generally understand. (Cutter and Viets 1964, p. 12)

Haste and compliance bear out in this description of the male physician's ability to "give quicker relief" and in the description of women as "childish" and without "greater presence of mind."

Time and haste in delivery remain two elements of American birthing practices evident in the role time plays for decisions about inducing women and artificially beginning labor. In Henci Goer's pivotal book *Obstetric Myths Versus Research Realities,* Goer builds the case that sonographic and clinical weight and date estimations are often wrong in determining due date, most babies deemed postdate are not postmature, and there is no evidence that routine induction at any gestational age improves outcomes (Goer 1995).

What potentially drives artificial induction of women? Being post 42 weeks can be a reason for labor induction. While prematurity is a serious concern for infants, the flip side of postmaturity appears relevantly insignificant. Prematurity is defined as being born more than 3 weeks before the due date, typically prior to 37 weeks, and according to the CDC in 2012, "preterm birth affected more than 450,000 babies—1 of every 9 infants born in the United States and preterm-related causes of death together accounted for 35 % of all infant deaths in 2010, more than any other single cause" (Center for Disease Control 2014). There is extensive evidence that premature birth of babies can cause short-term and long-term health problems, depending on the number of weeks short in gaining maturity and babies' birth weight. The same concerns for postmature babies do not exist and one potential reason is the inaccuracy of due dates.

The medical research literature points out that all clinical dating methods have a margin of error, some up to 2 weeks, resulting in a woman's due date being at best an estimation (Goer 1995). If there is a difference in accuracy between dating from last menstrual cycle and a first-trimester ultrasound, the American Council of Obstetrics and Gynecology (ACOG) recommends redating if the difference is more than 5 days when the ultrasound was done prior to 13 weeks and 7 days when it was done after 13 weeks (ACOG 2014). Clearly there is a considerable margin of error allowed for estimating the due date.

Women in this study consistently refer to their due dates, not their estimation dates, and the due date "passing" was viewed as significant:

> My due date was quickly approaching and I was so excited. I was so tired of being pregnant. And of course, was I on time? No. It wasn't until two weeks later my labor started. (Lisa, mother)
> My doula told me I very well may not be on time but I still wanted that to be the day. I had waited so long. (Karyn, mother)

Since the due date was estimated at 40 weeks after conception, these women going into labor "later" was disappointing to them but well within a reasonable timeframe. Time, pinpointed to a due date, was clearly viewed as significant for these woman and they reinforced the due date as an important measure in childbirth. The due date was on their calendars, shared with everyone, highly anticipated, but rarely met. The result for these women was a sense of disappointment at being "overdue" and a sense of "when is this going to happen?":

> Due dates used as a measure in childbirth is rather puzzling. Due dates are created by estimating 40 weeks after conception. Babies less than 37 weeks cause concerns, yet the reality is that 40–42 weeks is considered the range for ideal development and overdue babies are those born after 42 weeks. Yet we tell women, here's "the date." Does that make any sense? It really sets women up for disappointment in my opinion. And we are constantly working against that. Saying, it's just an estimate, you may go weeks past your due date, you aren't overdue, you are not a library book! (Sarah, doula)

The idea women have of being "overdue" only comes by establishing a sense of when they are "due" and thus setting up an imposed time that eventually works against them if they are not "on time." Time, measured in days or weeks, has relevance to the medical provider but doulas questioned how much to emphasize this for the mother. Doulas preferred to emphasize bodily markers that labor was beginning such as baby dropping, water breaking, back pressure during contractions, contractions that do not change with position changes, loss of the mucus plug. These were *embodied* markers that childbirth was close as opposed to focusing on a particular calendar date.

Birth as Embodied Time

The birthing event as depicted by the doula in both formal and informal interactions with women followed an embodied sense of time. The time that doula participants spent with their clients was rarely constrained by something other than the client herself. For example, in the prenatal and postpartum periods, doulas had several meetings with clients, either in their home or informal locations. Doulas' prenatal and postpartum visits with clients did not adhere to a predetermined sense of time set by a clock. The doulas in this study often entered the interaction without regard to how long the interaction might last and noted that they spent between 60 and 90 or more minutes with each client at each meeting:

> There really isn't a clock when it comes to my work. Except when I see what time it is I am driving to a house in the middle of the night (laughs). Then I am reminded of the time (laughs). But, in seriousness, my time with moms is really dependent on what they need at that point. I've had 30-minute meetings and two-hour meetings. (Jennifer, doula)
>
> She comes to my house, we sit and have tea and talk. The next thing I know time has just flown by and I have to jump up and pick up the dogs or something else but the time we spend is so special because it's just us and we talk and there isn't anything else to do but talk about whatever is on my mind at the time. (Amy, mother)

According to Jennifer, the amount of time spent with her clients "really depended on what they need," and for Amy, it revolved around "whatever was on [her] mind" as a mother. Debora explained how during her meetings with clients, she had particular questions that she wanted to address but most of the meeting time was "based upon the woman's agenda." For Debora, the woman set the time parameters:

> What stands out to me is that doulas are different because we don't have an agenda- a calendar filled every 15 minutes with clients. Not that I am not busy running from one client to another, teaching classes, going to births or more trainings. But the rigid timeframe doesn't work for me and I actually think moms really appreciate that. We are on the mom's agenda. Other care providers may have to get women in and out to see the next client or have a set amount of time they can spend but that's not what works for me. We sit and have tea and it almost seems decadent to the mom and then she feels like she is being cared for. That care is really about the time you spend with someone.
>
> I never want her to feel rushed. I never want her to think that there is something else more important at that time than her. And sometimes that is hard because I have a list in my head and I have to run here and there and sometimes it takes me saying, no, be here in this conversation, stop thinking about the guy that just cut me off in traffic. Just be here with her. (Megan, doula)

The lack of rigid timeframes was not only a way to set apart the doula as a care provider but also a means to potentially understand what makes doula care different; the amount of time dedicated to the woman and, as Debora would say, time devoted to the woman's "agenda." The woman, her body specifically, determined the time spent together.

Birthing women in this study explained that one difference in hiring a doula was having someone they could "call on anytime," someone who they "call whenever [they] had a question." Women participants, in asserting they could "call on their doulas anytime," suggested that the doulas' availability stood in contrast to their other care professionals, who were not available "anytime." The time that doulas spent with their clients was not restricted by a notion of an official business time, such as office hours; something which doulas suggested made it difficult in navigating the rest of their lives.

Within the birthing event itself, doulas depicted time as fundamentally in opposition to the medical typification of monitoring contractions using minutes. Because both the medical and the midwifery models are responsible for the clinical management of the birthing event, time measured by a clock does become a factor in clinical responsibilities for assuring the birth is progressing, for the health and well-being of mother and baby.

According to participant doulas, time measured externally, such as by a clock, had less bearing upon their role. They described that with every birth, it could be a 10-hour or 3-day event and they had no control over how long the process would last. Ultimately, because doulas have no responsibility to clinically manage the birth, following time was unnecessary beyond time between contractions. Instead doulas measured time experientially:

> I've had births were I arrived at night then went home at night and I missed two days so there is no set timeframe. (Kristy, doula)
>
> It's easier to not look at your watch- beyond timing contractions. If I look at my watch it means that I am thinking about something else and not the mother and where she is in the process. (Heather, doula)
>
> We are on the baby's timeframe and what time it is on the outside of the womb really has little bearing on what is happening. Time can distract you from being in the moment. (Laura, doula)

Time, as measured by a clock, according to doulas could actually be a distraction away from the attention at hand in the experience.

Doula participants often described "birth time" as something different than "normal time." "Birth time" is not structured like chronological time, for the focus is drawn upon "the moment," upon "the immediate," without the recognition that the moment has passed or another moment is coming. It was described as a "continual moment" of "being with the woman," in which the doula did not focus upon what has just happened or what might happen. Instead, the doula participant described staying in the perpetual moment and likewise encouraged the birthing mother to stay in "birth time" even when "normal time" interfered.

For example, Jackie (doula) described how the birthing woman and her partner could get "drawn into" watching the contractions on the monitor, or looking at the clock, which "draws the woman away" from the actual birthing moment:

> I saw them constantly looking at the monitor. It was like they were watching television and those lines were somehow mesmerizing. They just got drawn into that monitor until the women can't watch anymore because her body says "that's enough, I need you here with me." (Jackie, doula)

Being drawn away from the birthing moment meant, according to doulas, that the woman has time to think about what has happened, potentially feel bad about a decision, think about what might happen, or potentially feel like the labor is not progressing:

> I often hate the clock. It seems like it works against us so much of the time. The mom asks 'how long have I been at such and such stage' and then there is some judgment about that time. The mom thinks 'its been 2 hours and I am still at this stage!' Then the mind starts working to figure out why. 'Why has it been this long? What's wrong? And the spiral goes on from there. Let the medical team track the time but let the mom just be in that moment and keep moving forward without her stopping to make judgments about time. (Megan, doula)

In fieldnotes taken during an observation of childbirth, the role of the monitor and the timing of contractions become evident:

> The doula is trying to help her re-focus now that we are in the hospital. Laboring at home she had a rhythm and the doula, husband, and woman were all into a pattern- stopping during contractions, focusing together, after contractions relaxing. Now it seems to have changed. Husband and woman seem distracted. They aren't looking at each other or as close as when they were at

home. They aren't huddled together as they were in the home. Woman looks at monitor a lot during contractions. Husband starts looking at monitor. Husband asks 'how do they look' referring to contraction on monitor. Doula asks woman to look at her and listen to her voice. She talks about visualizing the baby. Doula tells the husband 'I'd like her and you, both of you, to try to ignore the change in surrounding and get back to getting into her birthing space.' Doula tells husband to focus on woman and not at the monitor and talks to the woman about focusing on a breathing technique. (Fieldnotes)

Time, or the clock, was often a distraction for women, according to doulas, and that distraction moved them out of an embodied moment, away from the experiential awareness of birth.

Doulas in this study also described the backward (what just happened) and forward (what might happen) reflections that can occur when a woman was not in the "moment" as detrimental to the birthing process. According to Heather, when a woman was taken away from what she was doing at the moment, during labor, she needed to be brought back to the most important place of concentration, the immediate moment. "This is not to say that birthing women do not need distractions" when they are too consumed by what is happening in the moment, according to Susan. She described using "distraction" specifically in regard to pain. But Susan defined the use of "distraction" as something that still kept the woman in "her own birthing moment," not a moment that is constructed by another person or a clock.

Megan (doula) portrayed birth as "entering into something that is entirely somebody else's space and time." She suggested that doulas entered into a "birth time" that was not their own time. Most importantly, Megan described the "birth time" that doulas entered as something that was not theirs to control or directly influence:

> Birth leaves all time behind and it is sort of all you're doing.... Women say that they have no idea if it's day or night outside. They'll say, "What time is it?" And I'll say 6:00 and they don't know if it's 6:00 in the morning or 6:00 in the evening. They go into labor and it's raining and they have their baby and it's sunny outside and they have no idea.... It's a space of really intense attention on what's happening. And my job is to hold that space and to do whatever I need to do to make that space be what they need it to be. (Megan, doula)

The woman's body dictated birth time and was unpredictable, so doulas saw time as resigned to follow the woman's bodily process. Embodied time in this sense exists beyond the confines of linear and temporal measures, and progresses without regard to even the rising or setting of the sun.

In describing the change from "normal time" to "birth time," doulas used phrases such as "stepping into another world," (Jennifer) or "being sucked into a moment that at times seems to never end" (Debora). The "birth world," according to Allison (mother), was one that began "with the clock," but that "clock quickly disappeared when you are really in labor." The time that transpired during labor at one point "may seem eternal" but then "you forget about even thinking 'what time is it?'." Amy (mother) explained how she "remembers having no idea how long [she] was pushing" and Julie explained how she thought it curious that she doesn't remember her daughter's time of birth:

> I guess it seems funny that I don't know what time Lilly was born. I mean, even now I would have to go check the birth certificate. It has never really seemed like something that important. I guess there are so many memorable moments that I remember, like what it felt like to push her out or when she started nursing. The actual time it happened doesn't quite seem that important to me. (Julie, mother)

Time in all of these instances was something external to the experience that was unfolding, and measuring or tracking that time became less important to focus upon.

Paula (mother) shared a copy of her birth story that her doula wrote up and gave to her during her (doula's) last visit:

> Sitting in the tub your high pitched tones made transition seem eminent, you were so close to having your baby and Stephen was pouring water over your back.... You became very focused with a look of intensity; it was time to start pushing.

These short examples reveal how Paula's doula used bodily descriptors instead of traditional time markers. Instead of noting mechanical time within the story, bodily changes (vocal tones) and emotions expressed (intent focus) marked the transitions in the birthing process. Paula's doula employs an embodied account of the birthing mother.

Mechanical time was characterized by doulas as the use of external measures, such as clocks or monitors, representing a technological imposition upon a naturally occurring and embodied event. According to participant doulas, mechanical time was not an appropriate measure to use in doulas' support role in childbirth. Embodied time, as described in the following examples, offered a much closer and more accurate measure of what was happening to the woman during birth:

> You can see on a woman's face when she is having a contraction. You don't need a machine to tell you. You can see the wave begin and fade by looking at *her* [emphasis added] not the machine. And when everyone sits staring at the monitor, looking away from the woman, the woman's body is not center, the woman is not center. Those moments should be focused on that woman and her body. (Debora, doula)
>
> 'Do you hear that difference?' Doula asks to husband. 'We are nearing transition' doula says to husband. (Fieldnotes)
>
> Every stage of labor is completely evident when you actually watch women give birth. You see their behavior; you see their faces, hear the sounds, the vocalizations, and see the sweat or blood. You see and hear transition and while the woman doesn't see or hear it you do because *they* [emphasis added] tell you, not in words but by their actions. (Heather, doula)

Moving from one labor stage to another was not marked by external time passing but rather by bodily signs. The clues of where a woman was in the process were all evident by centering on the woman herself rather than on clocks or monitors.

Doulas in the study depicted the progression from pregnancy to the birthing event and then into the postpartum with embodied qualities of time, as measured with attributes internal to the birthing woman, not with an external device. Laura regarded the use of mechanical time as something that constricted, not necessarily assisted, women during labor. She explained how in measuring time with external measures, such as constant electronic fetal monitoring, the natural progression of labor was often overlooked. She explained that while the use of technological measures serves "important purposes," the constant reliance upon the electronic monitor created an artificial sense of the labor progression:

> When labor doesn't progress as expected, when contractions stop or slow down, and then everyone looks to the monitor? Even the woman in labor? That tells me we are forgetting that birth happens to women, not machines. (Laura, doula)

In Laura's description, the monitor became not only the source of information about the labor process but was also relied upon to assess how the labor would progress. Laura reiterates how doulas view birth as central to the woman and her bodily signs as well as a concern that attention to external monitors of time takes attention away from the laboring woman, which should be the focus.

The Embodied Space Surrounding Birth

Birth requires a complex articulation of experience that is not available to the natural sciences, with their predisposition for relying upon visual articulations that yield the raw elements or data necessary for the production of knowledge (Grosz 1994, p. 97). Natural science relies upon epistemological theories grounded in observational knowledge that presupposes the neutrality of subject and disengaged object unaffected by the knowing process (Code 1991). However, within social science, the hegemony of positivist research has been combated with theories recognizing active, creative, cognitive agents (1991, p. 21). As the natural scientist measures the instigation of birth as timed intervals of contractions and the end of birth with the delivery of baby/placenta, the social scientist may measure the instigation of birth as the woman's recognition of a transition in her mental/physical state and the end of birth as the recognition by the woman of her new role as a mother.

The social scientist relies upon units of experience that are in themselves units of meaning (Gadamer 2004). Doulas approach childbirth from the perspective of a social scientist, in their belief that all women may not view childbirth in the same way, that women's bodies are active agents in the process that should take primacy, and that mechanical time is an external and often imposing measure upon birth. Doulas recognize the experience itself, not just the outcome of the baby, is a meaningful and necessary outcome.

Privileging the Experience of Childbirth

Experience is most often understood as the acquisition of knowledge or wisdom usually acquired through formalized systems and material texts, as primarily adopted by formal institutional education. This conceptualization preferences cognitive knowledge and formally developed understandings. Much like the process of dying, birth marks a bodily experience that is not easily articulated with the limited notion of experience available to natural scientists. Alternatively, experience can be understood as phenomena unique in context, what Gadamer describes as *erlebnis* and what can be referred to in childbirth as the *experiential* and *embodied* birth.

The *embodied* experience attempts to capture life (*leben*) manifesting itself in the experience (*erlebnis*) (Gadamer 2004). Yet all experiences are not necessarily *embodied* experiences. One can imagine moments where one is alive and other moments where one is "living life." Can you imagine walking through the motions of an experience but not feeling like you are living the experience? This is the difference between being alive, an outward appearance of the physical signs that one is alive, and living, the introspective awareness on the holistic cognitive, emotional, and physical interactions that come together when we are living life. This delineation of life and living represents the differentiation between experiences and *embodied* experiences that constitute themselves in memory as the lasting meaning that an experience has (2004, p. 66).

Embodied birth experiences manifest a reversal of control in which the phenomenon of childbirth takes over the person (the mother) and she is not merely a player in the process but becomes the process. In an *embodied* birth experience, time, space, and sequence are not determined by the participants, but rather by the process. In this study, birthing women, and those who labor with them, recognized the futility of attempting to control the time or the progression of the labor. Doulas especially recognized this as they attend many hospital births:

> I attend both homebirths and hospital births and one of the biggest differences is the pressure of time. Once you hit the hospital you are on the clock, if you haven't progressed in so much time you get the pressure for intervention, "you're only at this stage and we'd like you to be progressing faster," strip membranes, break water, start Pitocin, "if you want an epidural you should get it now or there won't be time later." It feels like a timed test with the clock ticking down. (Heather, doula)

In contrast to the time-driven experience of the hospital, doulas attempt to balance that with a focus on the experience to let the woman feel she is not alone:

The hardest thing you can expect a woman to do is somehow control what her body is doing in birth; primarily make it go faster. In hospital births you are watching the clock knowing that if she isn't at a certain place there will be an intervention soon but what I don't want is for her to know that. That's the team's responsibility to be thinking how is this progressing, what might we need to do if we seem stalled, make those suggestions. But she needs to be just *doing* the work. Our job is to keep all the pressure outside so she doesn't feel that. She can just focus on her work, her labor. We hold that place for her. (Debora, doula)

Holding the space, defined as the *embodied* birth experience, represented an invisible but bounded periphery created by doulas to allow the woman to be completely absorbed and involved in the experience of childbirth, to be within the process.

The embodied process of birth for doulas means allowing the body the same primacy of the mind and potentially challenging or questioning preconceived mental notions about birth to let the body dictate the process. Doulas described birth in a holistic manner with the unpredictable beginnings of labor, the distortion of time and space while immersed in the progression, and the unknown elements yet inevitability of the delivery of the baby. All this marks birth as a bodily driven experience, framing the argument that the woman's body must lead the process.

Doulas used specific language to challenge or reframe preconceived mental conceptions that some women had of childbirth to offer a view that the childbirth process must be one where the body takes priority over the mind and where the woman's body has authority. Doulas also used language to challenge commonly held misconceptions about breastfeeding and to redirect credit to the mother for the act of delivery. The examples below will be used to demonstrate how the language doulas used reinforced that childbirth was a process driven by the mother's body. Likewise, the assertions both women and doulas made that birth was uniquely feminine will be used to demonstrate how women viewed female birth support as important based on sharing the common experience of having the body of a woman. Both of these illustrations exhibit how doulas believe that the woman's body is both capable and central to the experience and doulas' work in childbirth is to support an embodied process that honors that belief.

The Embodied Language of Childbirth

Doulas used specific language to portray childbirth as driven by the body and therefore suggesting that women may need to set aside preconceived ideas about how it should unfold to let the body drive the process. Doulas often used specific phrases, in regard to breast-feeding or delivery, to challenge potential assumptions about childbirth in educational sessions as well as with individual clients. For example, doulas in discussing breast-feeding with clients consistently said, "when your milk supply increases," instead of the more common phrase, "when your milk comes in." The difference in language according to these doulas was important.

In both education classes and individual meetings, Doulas described the physiological reality of breast-feeding. They explained "women have colostrum, before the baby is even born" (Heather-doula) and "women have milk, as colostrum, ready from the first moment of breastfeeding" (Kristy-doula). Laura explained this physiological reality during a childbirth class and further explained how women are misinformed:

> They think they are waiting for their bodies to work, waiting for their milk to come in. This is simply not physiologically correct and really only makes women worry that they aren't able to feed their baby. Telling women, 'When your milk comes in…' basically suggests that women aren't feeding their babies. What a terrible feeling this passes on to women; that they aren't able to feed their babies. (Laura, doula)

The particular language used represents a belief by doulas that the woman's body is already able to feed the baby and represents an attempt to change preconceived ideas that women may have that their bodies "aren't working."

Doulas also consistently referred to "catching" as opposed to "delivering" the baby in education materials as well as in verbal interactions. Doula participants used this terminology to represent what the care practitioner, the obstetrician or midwife, does in the birth event. Heather explained that she used this terminology because she wanted her clients to "feel empowered." She suggested that using the term "delivering" gave the credit of childbirth to the practitioner and not the woman. Instead she preferred for "women to consider that they have delivered the child" and the practitioner was there "to assist in catching the baby."

While the use of alternative language may be considered trivial by some, the women in the study discussed how language was one way the doulas helped them reconceive the childbirth event. Mothers described how doulas gave them a "different" or "alternative" perspective upon childbirth that some had never considered. For example, Lisa talked about seeing breast-feeding differently after taking doula-led classes and the subsequent reactions she would encounter from friends:

> I actually found it hard to be around some of my friends during and after childbirth, especially when I was nursing. If I was nursing, they would say, "Are you going to nurse him here? Or are you going to cover up?" I would just say what Laura said in class, "He's entitled to eat, too." And one time I used her wonderful phrase, when I was beginning to nurse Sam. My friend asked if I wanted to go to the bathroom and I just said what Laura said, "Do you like to eat your lunch in the bathroom?" I guess I could have also said, "Do you eat with a blanket over your head?" (Lisa, mother)

According to Lisa, the language doulas used served to work against previous notions that her body should be hidden when she feeds her baby and she even took up that language when she was faced with friends wanting her to hide her body.

Paige described how from the beginning of her doula-led classes, she knew she was in the "right place." She described how the doula used the phrase "catch the baby" and her response to hearing that was, "oh yeah. That's what they [doctors] do, they aren't in the room long enough to do much more." In turn, Paige used the term "catching the baby" several times in her own interviews, representing how she had adopted this language. Paula also explained her adoption of the language used by doulas when she described how she would respond to her mother-in-law when she would ask about nursing. Paula's mother-in-law would say things like "Doesn't he ever quit? Can't you just put him down?" and Paula would respond with "as my doula would say, 'this is where he is supposed to be.'"

Language became a means for doulas to reconceptualize ideas of childbirth and breast-feeding to bring the primacy of the experience back to the woman's body. In both educative settings and also during childbirth itself, doulas depicted the process of birth as "letting the body take control":

> Doula says multiple times, 'this is your body working.' Doula says, 'this is normal its your body working to push your baby out.' Woman's shoulders tighten, her eyes close, her brow tightens. Doula says, 'you're tensing up, you are working against your body, let's visualize working with the contraction.' (Fieldnotes)

In labor, doulas responded to the nonverbal language from women and reminded them to focus on the bodily experience and bodily process. In the following interview excerpt, Paige reflected upon how her doula used certain language to help her through contractions:

> I really appreciated my doula's view of surrendering to the process. She would say "let go" and "just let this happen" and things that reminded me to let my body do what it is supposed to do, to not fight the process. I remember those words. They helped me relax into the process. And when I think back I think yeah, I was really fighting my body at times. But my doula recognized all that. She saw me tense and not letting go, so she reminded me. (Paige, mother)

Paige described having a conversation during her delivery. This conversation was not typical in the traditional sense of verbal interactions. First, Paige's body offered a sign that the doula recognized, such as tension, and the doula responded to it by saying, "let go." Paige responded mentally and physically with her body.

Paige explained how her birth doula picked up on nonverbal cues that resonated in the doula's understanding of birth, looking for nonverbal language from the body, and the doula responded by encouraging the mother to let her body lead the process. During childbirths, doulas pay particular attention to the nonverbal and physical signs, or embodied language from the mother. Doulas, because they spend a lot of time paying attention to the woman in labor, look for the woman's bodily language and respond:

> There is so much that is non-verbal. How the face looks, is it tensing, is it relaxed? What are her shoulders doing and how is she moving? Does she want you to touch her as a response or talk to her or both? We have to know those signs. Did the mom just tear off all her clothes? Is she grunting and *how* [emphasis added] is she grunting? Then she may be nearing or in transition. It's all about watching her. (Kristy, doula)

When Kristy states it is all about "watching her," she is articulating that a doula's techniques are in reaction to carefully watching what the woman's body is doing and letting the bodily signs dictate how the doula responds:

> Does she want to be touched? Does she recoil a bit—then that is not what she wants. Do her eyes look scared or nervous? I keep eye contact and reassure

her. Every birth is completely different and it's never the same process because it's never the same body. Even with a subsequent birth and the same mom it's still never the same birth. Her body is in a different place each time and I have to respond to that. But that's one of the things I love about my job. It's never boring! (Sarah, doula)

The woman's body in both of these examples is what doulas respond to during childbirth when they use particular techniques, and this represents doulas' view that the woman's body in labor holds primacy.

Letting the woman's body drive the labor process is reinforced by the language doulas use in interactions. Doulas specifically advise women to visualize the baby moving and reinforce working with the bodily movements, but also the technique of vocalizations during childbirth, in which doulas mirror the woman's vocalizations during contractions:

> She pressed the acupressure points on my shoulders, while bumping me up and down on the birth ball.... That's when I felt really sick and puked my heart out. And that was THE moment the actual labor started. I lost the sense of time and space, I didn't care I was completely naked, I was so deep within, just following my instincts and letting my body do whatever it needed to do. The contractions came with almost no recess, I went in and out of the shower, and my doula massaged my back. I hung on my husband's arms, vocalizing in low tones, visualizing my baby going lower and lower, trying to relax my muscles through the pain of the contractions. That cooperation with my body was so amazing.... And soon I felt the need to push. I was in the shower and slowly bearing down. The pain was different now and it was so interesting. My midwife came in with a portable monitor, got the baby's pulse and checked me. "Full" she said (I knew it!!) and they took me out of the shower since the hospital didn't allow birthing in water. I hung on the raised head part of the bed and felt an unstoppable urge to push. I worked with my body, I did everything to its will, and it was amazing... suddenly I felt the head crowning, and the contraction wasn't painful anymore. On the next one I pushed, and the head was out, and a second after—my son was born. The midwife caught him behind me and handed him to me between my hips. I was holding my son and once again—came this amazing euphoria of a non-drugged birth, of having this little miracle in my arms. (Irit, Birth Stories 2010)

The story Irit shares from a web blog describes several elements of an embodied birth. First, she describes "losing the sense of time and space" and "not caring that she was naked." This was also a common description used by mothers in this study; a description of moving into a different place, "where I had no idea of what was going on around me" (Lisa-mother), and "it was the opposite of having an out of body experience—I was totally focused *in* (emphasis added) my body" (Paula-mother), and "I am pretty reserved but when I hit transition the clothes came off and I really didn't even think about it. I was just so focused on the labor" (Allison-mother).

Likewise, in Irit's description, she describes "working with her body." These words were very common across the data and were used in education classes, personal interactions, and during the childbirth event. The notion of "cooperation with my body" shared by doulas is an essential part of an embodied birth experience. Vocalizations, as Irit also described, were a common technique doulas used during labor to reinforce to the woman that she was not alone and she had people there working with her:

> I like to moan with women, those deep guttural moans that really help ease some of the pressure of contractions. But I don't moan to show her how, she is already doing that. Maybe if she starts going into the high pitched tones then I try to get her back to the low pitch moaning but I moan to let her know I am there. They can be so focused and in the moment and their eyes might be shut but hearing someone else working with her lets her know she has support. She has someone working right alongside her. (Lisa, doula)

Vocalizations with the laboring woman were a way for the doula to demonstrate their benefit during contractions but also a reminder that even when the woman's focus was completely on the process, she had support. Doulas wanted to help maintain the woman's focus on her body while also letting the woman know she still had someone right beside her "working right alongside her."

From the daily language used, the materials available in education classes, and vocalizations and other techniques in childbirth, doulas represented to their clients that the childbirth experience was centered on letting the body direct the experience.

Doulas Understand a Woman's Body

In a similar vein, Allison made the argument that birth was not only distinctively embodied but that the role of labor support was uniquely feminine. She asserted that a man could not offer this support as he was not a woman (and thus does not have a female body):

> And that's another thing that makes me so mad. This notion that men will get upset if they aren't part of the process. We don't want to offend our husbands by suggesting that we need something more than they can offer? I hate the Bradley method.... It basically says that men can be doulas and women only need their husband for support.... It removes what is uniquely a female process and removes all possibility that women need other women for support. What is wrong in suggesting there is some realm that men are not experts, that women know more about this than they do. What's wrong with saying, you just don't know what I am going through and I need someone there that does. It doesn't mean we don't love them or need them to be there for support as well, it just means that there is something they cannot offer in respect to birth. (Allison, mother)

According to Allison, the woman by virtue of her embodied femininity and having lived in that physical body was privileged to experiences that a man was not. Allison argued that the body and inherent bodily experiences rendered someone without a similar body unable to recognize and offer labor support.

It is important to note that this explicit assertion that a man could not offer labor support was unique in the data. However, the reference to the birth process as embodied femininity was common. For example, most mothers in the study made reference to needing someone to offer her support during her birth, specifically a woman, who had personally experienced birth. While male partner's inclusion was described as "wanting him there," no mother specifically referenced wanting another male, other than a partner, for support.

Kathryn suggested that there was a difference in having a female versus a male obstetrician/gynecologist. She related this similarity to the reason she ultimately chose a woman as a care provider:

> It's interesting because I don't remember making a conscious decision about having a midwife over an OB. I mean, I just remember thinking I should ask around about midwives.... I had an OB/GYN but I started asking around

about midwives. I guess thinking more about it I would say that I had never really had a lot of positive experiences with OB/GYN's. I always felt like a little girl when I was with a gynecologist, maybe it was because they were always older men, which made me feel uncomfortable.... Don't misunderstand, I have had three different gynecologists in my life and all of them were nice and generally fine doctors. But, it was always having this feeling of being uncomfortable. I guess all women feel that way about exams, right? Yeah, for some reason it's the seeing of this baldhead in between my legs, all the while trying to make small talk. "Yes, I finished my degree several years ago. Well, it was in marketing. No, I don't know if I will stay around here." Baldhead emerges with an "All-righty, we're done." I mean, I am still uncomfortable laying naked with my legs in stirrups and a woman on the other end, but it's quite different with an older man down there- really just about any man down there. (Kathryn, mother)

In Kathryn's story, she described how she felt with a male obstetrician/gynecologist, and for her, the level of comfort is different with a female care provider. She explained a notable difference when "that person between your legs is a woman." She was referencing a particular aspect of female familiarity in regard to female anatomy and potential disquiet in having a man in such intimate contact.

However, she also described a power difference when she stated that she always "felt like a little girl" with a male gynecologist, and while even an exam by a woman is still "uncomfortable," it's "quite different with a male." In American society, violence against women and girls is prevalent. National crime statistics tell us: "On average, an estimated 211,200 rapes and sexual assaults went unreported to police (between 2006 and 2010)" (Bureau of Justice Statistics 2012), "about 20 million out of 112 million women (18.0 %) in the United States have been raped during their lifetime" (Kilpatrick et al. 2011), and "in the United States, 83 per cent of girls in grades 8 through 11 (aged 12 to 16) have experienced some form of sexual harassment in public schools" (AAUW 2001). A woman's preference for another woman in personal care situations may also be a reflection of either a previous harmful situation or the underlying knowledge of the possibility for violence against women and a greater level of comfort with other women.

More prevalent in the data were examples where participants suggested that either having the same biology in common or the same childbirth experience in common was preferred, privileging the female in either situation:

> I love my husband and he was great because he understood that I wanted another woman there with me. He knew that if anything she could help him understand what I was going through. He has no idea what this is like and never will. (Amy, mother)
>
> He sees me in pain and wants to fix it or make it go away. Because he loves me and it's awful to see someone in pain. But she [the doula] sees me in pain and wants to help me get through it because that's what she did, all women get through it, and she knows coming through it is what we share. (Karyn, mother)
>
> While I would hesitate to say that a doula has to be a woman, I just wouldn't consider having any other male beyond my husband there to support me. I just don't think I would take the support seriously and might even feel a bit defensive if there were several men in the room directing me. What exactly do they know about how this feels? (Linda, mother)
>
> I think a male doula would have a hard time with credibility, not that a man can't offer sympathy or empathy but at the point when a woman is looking at you saying, "it hurts" and you say "I know but you can do this," I just think that wouldn't mean the same coming from a male that isn't your spouse. I may not share the same relationship that a partner does but I do share the same experience of giving birth and that does mean something. (Jackie, doula)
>
> Woman begins to bend down, she grabs her husband's hand and squeezes. He makes a quiet noise, like some pain from the hand squeeze. The husband says, 'I am so sorry, I know how much it hurts, but ...(doesn't finish sentence)' A loud 'uhhh' sound from the woman. In a low tone she says, 'The hell you do. You don't know how this feels. You can't, you can't ever say that again.' Later woman says 'I didn't mean it. I'm sorry.' Husband responds, 'no, that's okay. I will just keep telling you, you are doing a good job. I know that.' (Fieldnotes)

Doulas made very similar references to having a woman's body and how it "helped." Laura said that having a woman's body is beneficial because "I am familiar" and women "know I have been in the same position, literally, the same birthing position that they are in." Karyn also refers to childbirth as "what we share," implicitly referencing a bodily experience that is shared with women. In this study both doulas and mothers addressed that while the childbirth experience can be shared with male partners, the bodily experience can only be shared with other women.

Susan suggested it was also more than "just giving birth," but also "being a woman who has been with many women during the birth process." Likewise, Megan offered a similar assessment:

> Actually, a friend of mine just last night was talking to me about this.... What she said is that having her doula there, her partner was her hands-on person and he didn't say much just because that's him. He's just not a talker. But he was touching her and holding her and doing all that stuff. She absolutely couldn't have done it without him and she had her doula, which she said was like a disembodied voice, this like female voice who kept saying you can do this, you're okay. She said that if he had said that to her that she would have thought 'fuck you, you don't know.' He has not done this and would never do this and can't. (Megan, doula)

Megan then reflected on the fact that like her friend's husband, she has never given birth. She asserted that it is the female body that understands the process, even if that body has not actually experienced the birth process, articulating a notion that the experience of childbirth is understood most fully by having had the same experience or sharing the same anatomy:

> But I do sometimes think that when I say, "Now you can do this," that they're thinking, "But you haven't." And I think that's true on one level. But I also think it's true that there's something about femaleness that gets it about female bodies. I've been with enough women who have given birth that they trust me even though I haven't. (Megan, doula)

Megan described how "there's something about femaleness that gets it about female bodies." She articulated that having a physical body in common, specifically a female body, resulted in shared experiences. Ultimately these critiques, offered by the mothers in the study, are based upon the assumption that living in a female body offered privileges of embodied "women's knowledge" that could not be understood without having a female body. It was a shared experience, a shared bodily experience, which doulas and birthing women in the study used to describe their relationship.

Doulas working with their clients view the process of birth as embodied, allowing the body the same primacy of the mind and potentially challenging or questioning preconceived mental notions about birth to let the body dictate the process. Likewise, doulas noticed women's bodily signals, often nonverbal, and responded. Doula participants demonstrated how they focused upon the embodied signals that women give during birth. These signals include facial expressions, tension or relaxation in particular body parts, verbal sounds, and emotional signals. The ways in which the complete focus of each doula was on the woman and her body as she labored demonstrated how doulas in this study regard birth as an embodied process. The notion of childbirth, and specifically labor, as an embodied process also involves an understanding of how doula participants regarded time within the childbirth process.

Conclusion

Doulas in this study recognized that childbirth was a continuity of experience, as Gadamer depicted in describing how one experience taken out of the continuity of life is at the same time related to the whole of one's life (Gadamer 2004). Viewing the childbirth experience as one that is simply *an experience*, not connected to previous or subsequent experiences, does not represent the relationship of that experience to the woman's larger life story. The childbirth experience connects both backward and forward because it becomes integrated into the woman's holistic life experience. Jennifer explains how important the experience of birth is for a woman as it represents a new shift from individual woman to mother:

> Some women start class with an attitude of 'I just want to get through it' and I understand that. Its scary for first time moms and so much has built up about the pain, as if that is all there is in childbirth. But I try to help them understand it's not just something to 'get through,' that seems so negative. It's like 'get it over with' but that seems like not the best kind of attitude to have because this experience makes you a mother. It's actually absolutely beautiful. I think I cry at every birth and that's not something you just want to 'get through,' it's something you want to cherish. You go into this process and then come out a mother- that's huge! So it's not something to just get through. It's something to prepare for and embrace and work through and look back and say 'my body is amazing, I am amazing, look what I did.' It's an event that changes your life from here on out, why would you just want to 'just get through it?' I say, 'This is you becoming a mother, a strong woman and now a strong mother.' (Jennifer)

Likewise in a childbirth class, Heather uses a marathon analogy to explain labor but also how childbirth maps onto the woman's life story:

> So, I like to equate this to a marathon. I started running and decided to train for a marathon, but I didn't just go out and run a marathon, right? No, I trained for it. So, in some ways you can see this as something to work toward, you learn about birth, you make decisions about how to prepare, you practice relaxation techniques, you get things organized for new changes, you do all this preparation work. And the preparation work is important because its helps you. But, like a marathon, the training, it's not the same as actually running it. Right? So, that day is always different than any training day. And that's the day that matters, it's the day that is hard, and you think, okay, am I really going to do this? Was I insane to try this? But the gun goes off and there you go. Okay, childbirth isn't quite like that and the reward is *so much greater* (emphasis added) but bear with me here. You are in the moment, you are running, its hurts, you want to cry sometimes, you want to soar sometimes, you want to quit sometimes, but you keep going because honestly what else can you do? You're in it. But then its over and you look back and say 'I did that!' But here's the thing, you carry that race with you. Your life is now different; you aren't the same person when you started that race. You will look back on that with these memories of accomplishment. It changes you. (Heather, doula)

Jennifer and Heather both view the childbirth event as an experience that women will carry forward and believe the process of giving birth, the *embodied* and *experiential* birth, will then relate to the rest of the woman's life experience from childbirth forward because the woman then takes on a new role as mother and that role begins with the experience of labor and childbirth.

Here is where we see the connection of the *embodied* experience as fundamental to the philosophy and subsequent methods doulas used in childbirth. Doulas recognized that the *embodied* experience of birth would be mapped onto memory and subsequently integrated into the woman's identity as a mother. As a result, doulas recognized that the *embodied* experience of childbirth should be protected for women not only in the immediate needs of birth, but also for the woman's integration of that experience into her future life. Doulas saw their role in the childbirth event as providing both love and advocacy, protecting the *embodied* experience because doulas place the highest value on the *experience* of childbirth.

CHAPTER 5

Love and Advocacy in Childbirth

Heather's birth story reinforces what much of the clinical research suggests—social and emotional support provided by a doula benefit women in childbirth. However, Heather's birth story demonstrates the impact when social support is absent, the need for social support, and the magnitude of the effect when social support is provided:

> With my first son, my labor was induced with Pitocin. The contractions were long and intense, with almost no breaks, and they felt like a vise repeatedly being tightened around my hips and spine. An epidural to relieve the grinding, iron-fisted pain sped up my dilation but sent my baby into distress as the Pitocin levels were increased again and again. Through most of my labor, my husband and I were left alone, terrified and clueless about what to do. Several painful and frightening complications arose the few times [my husband] had to use the bathroom, leaving no one to hold my hand or help me respond when doctors and nurses told, not asked, me what they were going to do to my body. When it was finally time to push, we discovered that my son was in the occiput posterior position—head down, but facing my navel instead of my spine. Immobilized from the waist down, I had to push him out that way. His positioning broke my tailbone and led to an extensive episiotomy to prevent the broad bones of his forehead causing a tear to extend into my bladder. Those injuries took months to heal and stop hurting.
>
> When they put my son in my arms, he was healthy and beautiful, but I felt almost no connection with him. I wanted so much to be a good mother to him, but before long my lack of emotional response made me start to think I was a bad one. Two years later, when I was diagnosed with severe,

long-term post-partum depression, I finally verbalized to a friend that, as much as I loved and wanted my baby, his birth had felt like a rape. With that negative experience and my depression in our shared background, mothering him was hard and sometimes painful—and that made me feel even more guilty. What kind of mother finds it painful to take care of her child?

When I got pregnant with my second baby, I wanted the experience to be different. I switched to a doctor and a hospital with a reputation for supporting mothers, and through my prenatal yoga class, I found an experienced doula. She lent me books and articles that changed my entire way of thinking about birth. In this new approach, the pain of labor contractions was not a sign that something was wrong, but a sign that my body was strong and healthy and was doing the work necessary to bring my baby into the world; fear could slow or even stop labor, while relaxation, confidence, and a sense of safety could ease and speed it; and birth was something my body was designed to do safely, something that I could help to happen by letting go of my psychological need for control over the process. Those beliefs are very different than the ones instilled in us by popular culture, most pregnancy books, and even by our doctors. They are also crucial to having a positive experience with labor and birth, like the one I had the second time around.

That time, I went into labor naturally. Since I was already 4 cm dilated and 50 % effaced, I went straight to the hospital. My doula kept me company, walking and talking with me throughout the delivery ward while my husband (who'd just worked a 20-hour day) got four hours' sleep. When my contractions got too strong for me to walk, I stayed in the delivery room, alternately hanging from [my husband] or my doula and sitting on a birth ball with her massaging and encouraging me and him holding my hands and singing to me. I went to the bathroom on my own steam at about 7 cm. After that, time and language lost their meaning for me; all I really recall is contractions so strong I couldn't breathe through them, and flopping like a rag doll in between them. I did ask for an epidural at one point, but by then I was already 8 cm dilated, and everyone knew it was too late.

I was not thrilled when I realized I'd have to push with no anesthesia. For several contractions, I resisted my doctor's instructions, thinking, *Surely somebody can make this stop*. Then I had what I call "my buy-in moment": I realized that, short of being knocked out with general anesthesia or asking for a c-section with no medical indication, the only thing that would stop this was me pushing out the baby. I asked for a squat bar, and the doctor and nurses jumped to install it and help me get into the right position. After two or three pushes, the intense pressure in my pelvis remained unrelieved and absolutely still, as if it wasn't a living thing inside me but a stone.

"Something's wrong," I said. The room went silent as everyone looked at me. To this day I remember my doctor's eyes, lake-blue and intent, as she listened to me tell her what I could feel: "He's not moving down."

The doctor squatted and checked out what was happening. She straightened back up. "Okay, he's posterior, and he's stuck. So after the next contraction, you're going to get on your hands and knees to turn him around." Posterior. The same position my older son had been in when I pushed him out under epidural anesthesia. Now, though, things were different. Grasping for something to help me get motivated, I asked, "Hands and knees–is that the Gaskin maneuver?" Ina May Gaskin was a touchstone for me; the decades of midwifery experience detailed in her books had helped me enter into this new way of thinking about labor and birth. My doctor's face broke into an enormous grin. "Yes, it is. Are you ready?"

I was. With her coaching, the nurses, [my husband], and my doula helped me turn over, brace my weight on my forearms, and push my bottom up into the air. When the next contraction came, I focused all the force I could muster *up* into my raised bottom. A deep-throated growl came from someplace inside me, and I felt the tremendous pressure in my pelvis shift and release, and then a tight burning sensation between my legs. Gasps and cheers filled the room, my husband grabbed my arm, and my doula and the doctor shouted, "You did it! You turned him around!" In fact, everyone there had watched the top of the baby's head rotate 180 degrees and surge forward as he turned and crowned in one contraction—that's how powerful it was to push from the right position.

Less than ten minutes later, I was holding my baby in my arms and the pain was gone. I looked into his face and—well, the only way I can put it is that *I knew him*. We had gone through this together, just as we had gone through the last nine (ten!) months together, and nothing would ever change that. I didn't know it then, but the perspective I gained in his birth would help me stop blaming myself for my depression and start enjoying my older son as well.

That is what birth can be like. That is the kind of birth we can choose to have. Painful, yes; a strong labor contraction can force you down on your knees. But it can also change you, if you let it. It can give you perspective on the smallest things in life; it can empower you to trust your own decisions; it can show you how strong you really are, and the astounding accomplishments of which you are capable. My natural birth, unintended though it was, remains one of the best experiences of my life–right up there with seeing my oldest son's eyes light up when I smile at him. (Richmond Doulas 2012)

Socioemotional Support

Emile Durkheim's study of suicide rates was the first to articulate the health implications of social support (Mander 2001). Durkheim asserted that social support carried a functional role in integrating people, which in turn had an impact on their mental health (Durkheim 1951). Early works defined support as either psychological or social (Elbourne et al. 1989), with social support defined as "intentional human interactions that involve one or more of the following elements: affect, affirmation, and/or aid" (Tarkka and Paunonen 1996, p. 71). Support has also been combined to cover psychosocial support (Wheatley 1998), while also referred to as emotional support (Thoits 1982). Emotional support has been defined as emotionally sustaining behavior, often in the form of listening, which serves to demonstrate a personal concern and personal intimacy (Gottlieb 1981) or as a sense of aid and security during stressful events that lead a person to believe that they are cared for (Cutrona and Russell 1990).

The notion of social support has largely remained ill-defined and vague, especially when not defined within a particular context. However, there is an extensive body of literature defining and articulating the benefits of social support in the health care setting and examples of how social support has been defined and articulated in terms of benefits in childbirth. Miller and Ray (1994) argued that the effects of emotional support are based primarily upon continued and long-term care. Social support has been found to have an impact on both the stress and the adaptation of individuals in health care settings (Spitzer et al. 1995) while creating a mediating effect on the participant's control over circumstances. This is in contrast to earlier views that support served as a buffer during demanding experiences (Cobb 1976). Sarason et al. (1990) found that social support reflected the individual's interpersonal relationships and the meanings attached to those relationships. While preexisting relationships offered the most likely influence in support, a history of conflict in those preexisting relationships potentially renders support ineffective (1990). This chapter supports this notion that a continuous support relationship, one that was viewed by the mother in terms of caring and love, was highly meaningful to women in childbirth.

Previous research on midwifery support in labor suggested that midwives have not been involved to the extent that women had anticipated. Spiby et al. (1999) found that "birth companions achieved a level of involvement closer to women's hopes than that achieved by midwives" (Spiby et al.

1999, p. 388). Likewise, a study of father's support during labor demonstrated that male partners acted differently than female companions during labor. Bertsch et al. (1990) used time sampling to study the behavior of male partners as the sole source of continuous labor support, comparing the behavior of male partners to a similar time sampling of doulas (Delay et al. 1987). Bertsch found the male partners were significantly farther in distance from the mothers and talked and touched them significantly less than did doulas when the birthing woman was experiencing pain (Bertsch et al. 1990). Similarly, when Brooks et al. (1995) examined the behavior of first-time fathers compared with female relations or friends, the male partners did not immediately provide the same type of support that female family members provided, and male partners stayed physically farther from the laboring woman than the female relation or friend.

Much research has demonstrated that when women have a supportive person that specifically addressed their emotional needs, outcomes in the childbirth context were improved (Hofmeyer et al. 1991; Hodnett et al. 2012; Kennell 2004; Morton 2002). Hodnett et al. (2012) suggested that one of the most successful interventions for reducing labor pain and the length of labor was the continuous presence of a trained, experienced woman focused upon speaking words of encouragement, holding the woman's hand, walking with her, suggesting position changes, instructing, and reassuring the woman and her partner.

Heather' story reflects the power of social support—first, in demonstrating what can happen when it is absent. Heather begins her story describing her previous childbirth experience and holding her first child for the first time:

> I wanted so much to be a good mother to him, but before long my lack of emotional response made me start to think I was a bad one. Two years later, when I was diagnosed with severe, long-term post-partum depression, I finally verbalized to a friend that, as much as I loved and wanted my baby, his birth had felt like a rape. With that negative experience and my depression in our shared background, mothering him was hard and sometimes painful—and that made me feel even more guilty. What kind of mother finds it painful to take care of her child?

In equating her first experience to rape, Heather articulates the emotional reaction to her first childbirth experience, described as "being alone, terrified, and clueless" and "leaving no one to hold my hand or help me respond when doctors and nurses told, not asked, me what they were going to do to my body." Heather connects her postpartum depression with her childbirthing experience and explains that together those led her to feelings of emotional guilt. She then questions her ability to be a good mother when she asks, "what kind of mother finds it painful to take care of her child?" While not all women without labor support experience postpartum depression, for Heather, she felt her first childbirth experience was lonely, terrifying, and ill-informed, which impacted her subsequent emotional state. She states, "When they put my son in my arms, he was healthy and beautiful, but I felt almost no connection with him. I wanted so much to be a good mother to him, but before long my lack of emotional response made me start to think I was a bad one." Heather articulates what she perceives as the impact of the birth experience upon her feelings of motherhood; that she was a bad mother because she had difficulty making an emotional connection after childbirth. This narrative gives insight to the power of emotions during childbirth and the potential for long-term impacts for the mother.

Heather's story also gives insight into nebulous terms used in emotional support, such as "intentional human interactions that involve affect, affirmation and aid" (Tarkka and Paunonen 1996, p. 71). In Heather's story, she described her second birth experience using examples of learning from her doula that feeling safe can impact birth:

> I found an experienced doula. She lent me books and articles that changed my entire way of thinking about birth. In this new approach, the pain of labor contractions was not a sign that something was wrong, but a sign that my body was strong and healthy and was doing the work necessary to bring my baby into the world; fear could slow or even stop labor, while relaxation, confidence, and a sense of safety could ease and speed it; and birth was something my body was designed to do safely, something that I could help to happen by letting go of my psychological need for control over the process.

She also described the feeling of having a person continually aiding her in labor:

> My doula kept me company, walking and talking with me throughout the delivery ward while my husband (who'd just worked a 20-hour day) got four hours' sleep. When my contractions got too strong for me to walk, I

stayed in the delivery room, alternately hanging from [my husband] or my doula and sitting on a birth ball with her massaging and encouraging me and him holding my hands and singing to me.

Heather then noted the affirmation when she turned the baby on her own and "gasps and cheers filled the room, my husband grabbed my arm, and my doula and the doctor shouted, 'You did it! You turned him around!'." And Heather ends her story with an emotional reflection on the impact of her own experience.

> That is what birth can be like. That is the kind of birth we can choose to have. Painful, yes; a strong labor contraction can force you down on your knees. But it can also change you, if you let it. It can give you perspective on the smallest things in life; it can empower you to trust your own decisions; it can show you how strong you really are, and the astounding accomplishments of which you are capable.

In her final paragraph she includes the reader by using the term "we" and "you" as recognition that she not only intended to share her story and her experience but also hoped that it would impact others.

Each of these excerpts give a deeper understanding of what emotional support means to women; it involves a sense of safety, of continual care, affirmation that their body is working with them not against them, and a desire to share the importance of emotional support with other women. Heather's narrative about what it meant to her personally is comparable to the data collected for this study; both reinforce that meaningful social interaction is important for personal emotional well-being.

Women in this study experienced a different emphasis on childbirth, one that focused on the experience of the birth and on the woman's body as driving the process. Likewise, doulas viewed their role in the childbirth event as providing both love and advocacy, protecting the *embodied* birth experience because doulas place highest value on the *experience* of childbirth. As a result, doulas viewed the childbirth process as one that maps onto a woman's memory and is important as she transitions into motherhood. Doulas described the emotional support that they offered in terms of intimacy and of love, resulting in advocating for the woman's wishes during the childbirthing event:

Birth is intimate. It is powerful. It deserves respect and honor.

How do you hold the space in the midst of trauma?

Love (DTI Admin 2013)

In the following fundraising address, Laura articulated the notion that labor was not just another experience, but rather one that would be integrated into the life history of the woman:

> You might be wondering how training a former teen mother to work with pregnant teenagers and have her go with them to the birth and to help them for a time afterwards could have an impact on the prison population, or change anyone in turning to drugs or violence. I can give you a lot of different answers, and I'm happy to elaborate with studies and with statistics and authorities. But really the answer is very simple and can be summed up in one word: love. That's what this is really about. Let me explain. When you take a woman who is about to have a baby, and you show her that you care about her, that you will nurture her and help her to take care of herself during this transformation, you communicate that she is worthy of love. And in order for her to love her baby, she must feel worthy of being loved herself. You show her by your actions, by your compassion, by your understanding of her experience and validating how very hard it all is and how very magical it all is, that she can do this and that *this* (emphasis added) is how you love. What is parenting if not loving? And to expect someone who has had poor role models and has been told over and over again that she is a failure, and then we expect her to love her baby effectively and well? A woman who has been abused by the adults in her life and is now turning into those adults by virtue of becoming a mother; how can we not offer her the chance to learn? How can we not offer this baby the chance to come into loving, knowledgeable, healthy arms? (Laura, doula)

The recognition that the childbirth experience would be integrated into the lives of the mother fundamentally sets apart the role of the doula from other caregivers; the doula's role is to offer care, primarily love and advocacy, during the transition from childbirth into parenting because doulas believe that the experience of being loved and advocated for will be integrated into a woman's future life as a woman and mother.

Love

The use of the word "love" by both doulas and women cannot be understated. Love was a prominent theme in the data and used often by both doulas and women:

> My husband is in the military so he was overseas and [my doula] was what got me through it all. I ended up going early and I had my older son but without a lot of support. She was amazing, she made me feel that I could do this and I would look at her and think, 'yes I can do this. She's done it. I can make it through it.' She will always be a part of my family and a special place in my heart. I am so grateful for her and all this love we have. (Amy, mother)
>
> I felt loved and supported. I was so filled with joy and love, those are probably the best words for the entire experience. (Karyn, mother)
>
> As we pulled up to the emergency room I saw my doula and her apprentice walk up to our car. They helped me out and we started to walk through the doors of the hospital. While my husband was signing all the paper work for me I remember telling everyone I was so tired. Each contraction was still 2 minutes apart and every time I felt one start I would tense up. [My doula] started to talk me through them. She told me of all the women in the world that were laboring alongside me, some of them without any support. The words put it in perspective—I had 4 lovely individuals who were there for me. I was the lucky one. I felt [her] hands rubbing my forehead, I felt my husband's arms around me, I heard my mother telling me how proud she was. All these distractions were getting me through each one. I felt so loved. (Birth without Fear 2013)

It is important not to simplify the use of the word "love" that so prominently factored into the stories and language used by women and doulas. The notion of love, as doulas and women described, was rather complex. It was based on establishing intimacy in the doula–woman relationship, which required time in building trust with the mother. Yet the intimate relationship was a one-sided intimacy; one in which love was given to the woman but not relevant to be reciprocated. The love that doulas described as giving to their clients required a different approach to love than a partner or family relation; a detached love that could serve to advocate when the woman was immersed in the experience and may not be able to self-advocate.

One-Sided Intimacy

Doulas described a considerable difference in childbirth experiences with a client to whom they had a strictly "professional" relationship:

> By the time the birth comes I'm someone that they feel very close to and comfortable with. I have had clients with whom I have had much more of a professional distance and that just doesn't work as well because they're not as able to let go during labor because they don't feel comfortable. (Megan, doula)

Megan suggested in this excerpt that having a "professional relationship" did not offer the intimacy required for the client to "let go" during birth and "feel comfortable." Sarah (doula) explained how having a professional relationship with clients "doesn't allow for me to really help them." She explained that the birthing woman "never really gets comfortable with me, so it's not any different than having another nurse or medical staff in the room." Jennifer (doula) articulated the limitation of a professional relationship when she said "being comfortable in labor is all about trust. If a client doesn't know you how can they totally trust you?"

Interestingly, doulas in this study referred to themselves as labor support professionals and in the literature are referred to as paraprofessionals. Yet a "professional" relationship was not ideal. How might we understand this potential contradiction? The answer involves a greater understanding of what the relationship means between doulas and women; a relationship that requires intimacy, a very specific kind of "closeness to women" as described by mothers and doulas.

Intimacy for doulas in this study became manifested within the notion that they were part of the "woman's team," separate from hospital or other health care staff. The separate identification that the doula was part of the "woman's team" carried with it the notion that the doula was "closer to the woman and her personal needs and personal perspective" than any other health care member. Susan and Sarah both described the difference in being the client's support person as opposed to a hospital staff member. Sarah stated:

You're not in any way affiliated with the hospital services. That doesn't mean you can't work together with the nurses, that there's not a shared sense of support for the woman. But it's different because it's more constant, and it's more than being just supportive, there's a history there, a relationship. (Sarah, doula)

Susan suggested that while nurses can offer support, they are not prepared to offer what a doula can:

A nurse could technically do what I do. She could offer similar support but it is not the same. She doesn't, she hasn't had a relationship with the women. She hasn't spent time with her, listening to what she wants, knowing what is really important to her. There is a lot of knowledge that a doula has in regard to the woman's expectations and those expectations are important to recognize. (Susan, doula)

During an observed doula training session, Laura described how she physically supported women in labor. She also referenced her role as a "mom":

Where I stand physically in the room, how close I am to them or how far away I am from them, depending on what's going on, my language, my silence, attending to dimming the lights, answering needs before they're expressed, if I can. So, I do things like getting that glass of water ready for her, have a snack for him available, try to pick up on those nonverbal cues that she's getting tired or she has to go to the bathroom or let's get her up and walk her around. Just kind of move in, just being a mom, it's a lot of what you do with little children in your family. It's sort of being that emotional glue if he's spiraling out in anxiety and she's getting deeper into the labor and I kind of hold that together for them. (Laura, doula)

Each of these excerpts demonstrates not only a view that the doula played a different role in being on the "woman's team" but also that the care and support provided was longer-term care. Doulas established a relationship with their clients over many months, many meetings, and many hours. Because doulas in this study worked with clients before, during, and after childbirth, the duration of their time with mothers was significantly more than other care providers. The amount of time with clients and the way doulas focused on the woman's interests, as mentioned in the previous chapter, provide opportunities for doulas to learn about their clients and get to know them more personally. It is the personal intimacy that both women and doulas implicitly refer to when describing the doula–mother relationship.

Both doula and women participants made references to familial relationships, such as mother, sister, and the female body, denoting a level of intimacy between doulas and mothers. Every doula in the study made some reference to offering "womanly support," either explicitly or implicitly in their descriptions of their role in labor. It is not only doulas who suggest that labor support often took the form of a relationship comparable to mother or sister. The term "mothering the mother" predominates in the informational and advocacy literature on doulas, and both doulas and women used this term when describing their relationship with each other. However, the relationship described by doulas and birthing women participants did not always directly reference a motherly relationship.

Doulas also recognized that some women did not want their mothers in the labor room. "There can be a lot of relationship baggage" when a woman's mother is in the room, which some "women know will not be helpful in labor" (Jennifer-doula). Paige and Lisa both described how they specifically did not want their mothers in the delivery room. Paige said she "didn't want this to be about her, as it is in [their family] whenever there is a crisis," and Lisa said she "thought her mom would be too worried if [she] was in a lot of pain and really push having an epidural." Julie described how her mother had very specific instructions not to express any thoughts or advice directly to Julie, instead to express those thoughts to her doula.

Some doulas and birthing women referenced the relationship in terms of being "sisterly," "like an aunt," or a "really close female friend." The use of terms such as "sister," "aunt," and even "close female friend" implied the same qualities of caring, just within a different female intimate relationship. The use of the term "mothering" was not consistent across the data. However, the belief that the doula's role was an intimate one, producing a type of care different from other providers, was consistent across the study.

The care doulas provided represent a relational intimacy between doula and client. For these doulas, "giving women sips of water between contractions," "wiping blood as it runs down her leg," "making sure she has something to stand on so that she's not on the cold floor," or "reminding her partner that if he needs to go to the bathroom that he can," all encompassed elements of the physical nature of their practice. However, these "support" techniques also implied closeness to the woman.

One of the participating doulas, in noticing that a woman's feet would get cold standing on the tile floor of the hospital, took notice of small measures that would make her client more comfortable. Laura referred to these small measures as, "It's just like being a mom. You notice those things." Sarah reflected upon her memories of women in labor, "I remember women's faces, really close to women's faces. Stroking their hair, you know, speaking in their ears, holding their hands, being so very close." Laura and Sarah in describing their "physical support techniques" also referenced their relationship, their intimate relationship with their clients.

The physical closeness of doulas in this study to their clients mirrored the emotional closeness and a relational closeness of a mother to her child that doulas wanted to emulate. Doulas and mothers referred to "mothering" or "being mothered." As an explicit reference to denote a relationship between women, mothering was also implicitly evident in interactions between doulas and women. Attention to details in birth, such as "giving women sips of water between contractions," described taking notice of a situation in a way that implied a concern for another individual in the same way that having a relationship with that individual would imply.

In the same way, doulas had interactions and made changes in the labor environment that implied a concern for the woman, in a way that women participants internalized as personal and relational. Julie described in her birth story how she at times could not tell if the touch was from her partner or her doula:

> So, we tried our best to eat something and then go to sleep. By early morning I was going a bit crazy and told Henry to call our doula because I needed some encouragement because I was really feeling like things were beginning to move... She said to check in with my doctor, we did and after trying to talk through a few contractions he said I should make my way to the hospital. We called our doula and she was at the hospital waiting for us. She was there when I got out of the car and she and Henry were holding me through contractions as we made our way into the hospital. I have a very vivid memory of her holding my shoulder and then slowly moving her hand down my arm as my contractions faded. It made me feel more relaxed as the contractions ended and then Henry started doing something similar. It was amazing, at times I didn't know whether it was her or Henry but I remember that feeling so, just very caring. I remember hearing her breathe with me and focusing on our breathing together. Henry did that, too. I don't know if she told him to do that or if he just picked that up, I should ask him about that. (Julie, mother)

Julie articulated a relationship with her doula in her labor that was described as caring. However, nowhere in Julie's birth story or interview did she describe any other person, except Henry, in this manner. She repeatedly emphasized how her doula provided a different kind of care. She said:

> It was just so different in the way the nurses treated me than our doula. I was so surprised because I thought that I would have this amazing team in labor. And I mean a team that included nurses and doctor. Going in I really liked my doctor. But what happened was my team was really only Henry and my doula. Nurses were in and out, I don't really even remember the doctor... but the nurses were doing things for me, which was helpful. They might get me something and they were really kind, but it was Henry and my doula that were supporting me. I don't think it was like the nurses didn't care about me, they were so nice. But they just weren't the ones giving me support and being so close and ...and being so... really caring. (Julie, mother)

Julie appreciated her nurses and their kindness, but she described her partner and doula as considerably different. Her partner and doula cared for Julie in a different way. Julie's descriptions of how her doula "held" her and how it was "amazing" implied a sense of intimacy.

Reflecting a similar sense of intimacy, Debora described her interest in serving women as "maternal." She related that she had a "real interest in women, a genuine interest in their well-being, their pregnancy, and their babies." Sarah offered similar feelings of "nurturing women" as a reflection of not having close female familial connections in her own life:

> I guess maybe by doing doula work, one of the things I get back is, just by being able to give that real sweetness, that real nurturing, that real in some ways mothering of a women or a couple. It fulfills something I didn't have for myself and didn't have in my family so it's like filling that whole, that something that was missing. (Sarah, doula)

For Sarah, mothering was a way to view the birth process as an intimate one, by relating the support that she offered to a close female relationship. Likewise, Heather described the relationship she has to her women clients as intimate, but temporary. When Heather encountered previous clients she described an immediate bond or "connection with women."

This connection, according to Heather, resided in an intimate relationship, an "intimate closeness at an intimate time," both have shared with each other. However, as most doulas in the study suggested, the intimate relationship was not one that was maintained.

Laura, in identifying her role as a "mom," suggested that the relationship she had with the birthing woman reflected an intimate one in which she served a motherly role, "being the emotional glue" for the woman and her partner. However, according to Laura, that motherly role did not mirror completely the parental relationship. Laura described her mothering women as a one-sided intimacy:

> Mothering women is an interesting way to think about the relationship. Most of the time, if I've done a really good job, they really don't know who I am, and that's kind of how it ought to be. We're not going to be friends. It's that weirdness of a one-sided intimacy. (Laura, doula)

A one-sided intimacy is one that is not expected to be reciprocal. Doulas did not expect their relationships, even though intimate, to go beyond a client relationship. Again, what emerges is the conundrum of the professional yet intimate relationship. Mothers are clients and not expected to be "friends," yet doulas must know the woman and her wishes and be close enough for the woman to feel a deep level of comfort and trust at a point when a woman is at her most vulnerable, in childbirth. Doulas provide care that does not necessarily make logical sense. Their role is to become highly knowledgeable about the particular woman, build a high level of trust and comfort, treat her with the love and care that you would in an intimate relationship, focus on the experience as opposed to the outcome, and then end the relationship at a particular time. This seeming contradiction may be exactly what makes doulas effective and what makes replication and generalizations about doulas difficult.

Advocacy

According to doulas, their role implied to other caregivers that there was a woman in the room whose purpose was specifically to take care of the laboring woman. Participants noted that this role could be seen as problematic for other caregivers, specifically medical professionals that might envision the caregiving role as solely their own. For example, Paula described a nurse seemingly agitated with her doula:

> I think at one point I offended one of my nurses. She made a really quick comment like, "well, I thought she [referencing the doula] was going to be doing that." It was after I had delivered Sarah and I was in the bathroom and I pushed the button because I felt really weak in my legs and my doula was holding Sarah. I had asked her to be with her and I was in the bathroom. The nurse said I had to get up and go pee. She said if I didn't, I needed a catheter to empty my bladder. Then she left. So when in a few minutes I called for her help she made this comment like she was really busy and she thought my doula "would do that." So, what I wanted to say was, "what do you do for women who don't have doulas? Do they have to sit and wait on the toilet?" Later I was just thinking man, am I glad she wasn't there holding my hand during labor. (Paula, mother)

Paula's perception of the nurse being offended based on the nurses comment of "I thought she was going to be doing that" might suggest that nurses, seeing themselves primarily in the caregiving role, consider themselves displaced by the caregiving support being offered by a doula. Heather elaborates on this when she explained:

> Some nurses love us. They realize they can't spend the time with mothers like maybe they would have liked to. But then there are others that see us as interfering or maybe just taking up extra space in the room. But I do think there is usually a bit of tension when the mother wants to get advice from us or wants to hear a suggestion from us versus the nurse. Sometimes they [nurses] see the labor room as their domain and while fathers or family is okay, for some reason we aren't. (Heather, doula)
>
> I find that if we just do the physical support, the handholding or rubbing backs, the nurses are fine with that. It's when we remind them of the woman's birth plan or when the mom does something we suggest, that's when the nurses can potentially react. (Megan, doula)
>
> If we keep quiet then they are fine with that, it's when we assert something the mother asked us to that the nurses can get their nose out of joint. (Kristy, doula)

While Heather describes how partners or family members may not have a similar affect upon nurses feeling displaced, Megan and Kristy further explain that certain elements of their role are more acceptable than others. Specifically, doulas that engage with the nurse on the mother's behalf are viewed more negatively than the doula that just offers physical support techniques. Since doulas are recognized as labor support paraprofessionals and mothers specifically have asked them to fill that role, an implicit assertion is that the hospital may not be providing an element of care during labor, even though both doulas and women viewed the care provided by the doula as a fundamentally different kind of intimate care that would not be traditionally expected from medical staff.

One role of the doula is to advocate for the mother during labor when she may not be able to advocate for herself. Allison stated that she specifically wanted "her doula to maintain her wishes for an unmedicated birth even when she was asking for pain medication." Julie shared a similar request and explained why she wanted a doula with her in labor when she said, "I know the pain will overwhelm me and in the moment I will want something but that is *that* [emphasis added] moment and not what I really want my birth to be like." Mothers described wanting a doula present so they could maintain wishes they had for a particular birth experience and recognized that their family may not be able to provide that advocacy:

> I know [my husband] cant see me in pain. If I say I need an epidural he will jump to it. He hates to see me upset in general, I can't image what he is going to be like in childbirth when I am overwhelmed with pain. But what I want is someone to say, 'okay, lets give it a bit more time.' And not jump to medication. (Amy, mother)
>
> I want my doula to be the cool calm head in the room knowing what I want. I don't know if nurses even read birth plans and they certainly don't know how adamant I am about some things and what I can give up. I want my doula to remind me about what I intended multiple times and not jump the first time I get hit with pain. (Lisa, mother)
>
> I know the moment I go into labor everything I have learned will fly right out the door. I don't want [husband] to have to stop and think, okay what does that mean, what do I do now? I want her to remind us, 'okay this means this and let's try this.' (Paula, mother)

For these women and others in this study, the doula played more than solely a physical and emotional support role. The doula was expected to advocate for what the mother wanted during labor, specifically advocating to the hospital staff:

> My experience with [doula] was pretty much what I had hoped. Initially we were on the fence about hiring a doula and I kept saying, well, will it be worth it, mostly meaning the money but [my husband] finally said, look Linda, we have no idea whether this will be worth it but we really never know so let's try this. I think it will make you feel good to have a doula there so let's just try it for our first one. I think at one level I wanted him to just say that so then I immediately went into gear making calls and asking for referrals. It was awhile and at one point I thought, well maybe this isn't going to work out. I had talked to a few and we really hadn't jelled, I didn't seem as assured about themselves as I would have liked or they seemed to just, not follow my lead when I would ask questions… so I would say something like, 'I really want to have an unmedicated birth' to see how they responded and one kept saying, 'yes, unmedicated is great but, well if you want medication its okay to change your mind.' But that's not what I wanted to hear. I wanted someone with a lot of confidence in what I wanted. But then I got this recommendation to call [doula] and from our first meeting we really clicked and I knew she would be able to speak for me if I needed her to in the delivery room. When I said 'I really want to have an unmedicated birth,' she replied, 'then that's what we go for and I will try my best to help make that happen.' I didn't want someone wishy-washy, letting me change my mind with every labor pain. I wanted her to say, 'remember what you wanted? Remember your goal?' (Amy, mother)
>
> I am so glad I had [doula] there. When we got to the hospital my labor completely stalled. She reminded me that this happens and we were up walking and moving to get it going again. Then they put me in bed for monitoring and no contractions for about 20 or 30 minutes. So this is when the nurse started pushing Pitocin. [Doula] said 'well, first let's get her up and maybe lets walk a bit more' and got me up and moving again. I almost felt [doula] was running a bit of interference because it seemed like every time the nurse came in I was in the shower, or on the ball, or talking me through visualizations so she kind of kept me, like shielded, until contractions started up and then wham they really took off so Pitocin no longer was an issue but [doula] really helped me avoid that and get back into labor naturally. (Paige, mother)
>
> Basically I think one thing they do best is get the hospital staff out of your hair so labor can progress and you can get into your own space. All the interference from every time they want to monitor you can shut you down

so when the monitoring was done my doula would say 'do they look good? okay so lets move around some more.' (Julie, mother)

In these excerpts, mothers expected doulas to run interference with hospital staff suggesting certain interventions and helping give the woman more time to progress on her own. Not all women were explicit about wanting doulas to intercede when interventions were suggested, but all women expected their doula to know their wishes about the labor experience and actively work to help make those wishes a reality:

I had a crazy birth plan. I wanted particular music, low lights, just a list of certain things, no episiotomy, not to be offered medication -even though that happened several times anyway- and [doula] was the one making sure I was getting what I wanted. (Paula, mother)

Doulas, as intimately aware of the women's wishes, are then in the role to help facilitate those wishes being honored based on what is medically reasonable. Therefore, the doula must be able to offer a level of intimacy in care, as a family member would, yet also remain detached to also fulfill the role of advocate.

Detached Caring

Doulas described the advocate role as requiring a level of detachment even in the midst of very intimate caregiving. The level of care doulas described required a level of intimacy and closeness to the woman. However, the role also required the ability to detach from the intimate caregiving role to both understand and potentially interpret the broader event:

I remember vividly one experience when we were fairly early in labor and we were working through a contraction when the labor delivery nurse walked into the room very casually saying, "We lost the baby." Of course what the nurse meant was that she lost the signal from the fetal monitor. She was watching from the nurses' station and the monitor had lost the signal. And it was easy for me to understand what she meant by the nurse's casual tone and by her relaxed nature that she really meant that she lost the signal from the monitor. If something was wrong, she would not be so casual. Five people would be flying into that room if there was something dire happening. However, at the same time I knew that that is *not* (emphasis added) what the mother was hearing and that was confirmed when I saw her face. She looked terrified. So I knew that what the mother heard was that the baby was dead. I immediately turned to the mom and said, "They can't read the signal on the monitor, the baby is fine, they just need to rearrange the monitor." But for that brief moment that mom was in shock. (Laura, doula)

Laura's experience as a doula allowed her to see the situation from multiple perspectives. Laura recognized both what the nurse intended with the comment "we lost the baby" and how the mother interpreted the comment as "the baby is dead," which was confirmed on the mother's face. Her ability to assess the situation and what was happening required the ability to detach from the physical and emotional work of labor support to understand and interpret the situation.

Doulas both demonstrated and described the need to be a more detached caregiver:

> Sarah remained focused on [the mother] during the entire contractions. Her eyes never left. [The husband's] eyes would go back and forth between [mother] and monitor. Nurse enters room during a contraction and attempts to talk to [mother]. [Husband] looks to nurse to say 'hold on a second.' Only when the contraction was over would Sarah break eye contact to look at or respond to the nurse. As labor progressed [husband's] eyes stayed focus on [mother]. As [husband] maintains eye contact and focus, Sarah is able to talk to a nurse during a contraction asking for information and heart tones. Sarah asks nurse if monitoring could end so [mother] could get out of bed and into a bathtub. [Mother] didn't ask to move but appears relieved to be moving and says 'that feels better' when she gets into the bathtub. (Fieldnotes)

In this example, the doula begins very focused on the mother, potentially as a way to model to the father to keep eye contact and a focus on the mother. As the father takes up this role and then maintains his focus on the mother, the doula then asks the nurse for labor information and then makes a request on behalf of the mother, a request she never verbalized to the doula but potentially a previous request made in a birth plan or during a prenatal visit. Sarah was not only a focused caregiver but also a detached advocate to speak on behalf of the mother.

Doulas describe a level of detachment necessary to do the advocating portion of their role:

> I have to be the calm and level head in the room. I have to look calm even if there might be reasons for me to be worried. I don't want the mom to see

worry in my face because that worry might be completely unwarranted. She has to be focused on her labor and not what might be going on, unless she absolutely has to address a concern. (Sarah, doula)

During labor the woman goes to a different place. I know that sounds strange but any woman, especially those working without any medications, will say the same thing. That everything stopped and they just *were in* (emphasis added) labor. So, we can't expect women to think rationally at that point. They just have to be doing it, they can't pull out and stop and think, should I or shouldn't I do x or y. There needs to be someone there saying, okay, we may need to get on hands and knees or she needs counterpressure here, or remember she didn't want an IV, is an IV medically necessary right now? If there are questions to be asked, someone that can pull away and ask them, then listen to the answer, is what we can do. We have the experience to understand what normal births look like and can ask those informed questions and then go back and explain what is happening. In such an intense time we can't expect the mom to navigate all that for herself and likewise dad should be just as focused on mom. (Jennifer, doula)

This might be their first time or third time but we log so many births, we've seen so much that we bring that experience with us to every birth. We can keep calm because to us it doesn't look like chaos, we are used to birth. Blood, vomit, crying, all that looks normal so we aren't stressed. Not to say that we don't get frazzled at times or when things escalate and might be thinking "uh-oh" but we have to keep the level head for them [the parents]. (Megan, doula)

The role of an intimate yet detached caregiver was also seen as a particular challenge by many doulas, especially when wanting to uphold the woman's initial wishes prior to labor while women were in the midst of actual labor:

That's such a tricky piece to our work, how much to we push back when women say now they want medication. I always go through this mental game in my head. Does she really want me to go get the nurse for an epidural? She was adamant before about not wanting one. I want to respect what she asked me to do but then the nurse is looking over me probably thinking, you are keeping this woman from getting relief. But [the nurse] wasn't there during all our meetings and discussing what those options were and listening to the woman saying, 'no I want an unmedicated birth, I know what medication does to my body or the baby and I don't want that.' Then labor hits and now she's in pain and I am the one saying, 'wait, let's give it more time.' I have to be the 'bad guy' kind of but only because she asked me to do that- to question her to try to keep her unmedicated. (Debora, doula)

[The mom] says to me, 'I didn't mean it, I want drugs.' So [the husband] and I stop and we don't really respond for about a minute and she says again, 'I changed my mind I really need something, please.' And she really emphasizes the please to us. She is looking at us pleading. So I look at her direct in the eye and say, 'you are doing this, you are doing amazing.' [The husband] looks a little sheepish and I just look at him and say the same thing, 'she's doing this.' But the whole time I am thinking, 'okay, is this the pain and [the mother] or maybe just the pain? I decided to say, 'okay let's get through just a couple more together.' I felt like she was really close to transition and maybe just a bit more. We had all these conversations about medication and she was very firm to me about having an unmedicated birth. But maybe she's farther away than I think and a chance to rest would be exactly what she needs. You don't know. No one really knows. The nurse comes in and checks [the mother] but she never says anything to the nurse so I am thinking, 'she's not asking the nurse. Do I bring it up? [The husband] is silent and he doesn't' say anything.' A few minutes and transition hits and she never asks again. Did I do the right thing? Later [the mother] said, yes, 'thank you for not listening to me' but it's such a challenge in the moment because [you know] how she feels *and* (emphasis added) you know what she wanted. So you are balancing those things in your head. (Megan, doula)

Doulas address the difficulty of balancing women's previous wishes with labor realities and question how much they should push back, even when the woman has asked them to, or follow the immediate wish for an intervention.

Doulas, like in Debora's previous excerpt, recognize they are criticized for promoting their own agenda of unmedicated childbirth at the expense of women's own wishes for pain control:

In general I think doulas promote natural and unmedicated childbirth. Let's be honest there's just too much information that one intervention leads to another and labor progressing naturally and ending without drugs is just better for mom and baby and breastfeeding, bonding, etc... Does that always happen no- but that doesn't mean as doulas we can't outwardly support what we know. It doesn't mean we have an agenda beyond wanting to see women given all the information to make informed decisions and striving for a natural and unmedicated birth in a normal or low-risk pregnancy. (Kristy, doula)

I never want a woman to feel bad about any choices they make in labor. If they go in saying no drugs but then they get an epidural that is their decision. I'll say, 'that's was a good decision' even if I thought, maybe if she gave it a bit longer... it's not my job to judge her, it's my job to support her. If she has specifically asked me to help her not have medication I will do my best but in the end all women need to feel they are strong and accomplished. We don't need women critiquing themselves as mothers the moment they become one. (Heather, doula)

According to these doulas, the critique of "having an agenda" was more likely attunes to the woman's agenda of going into labor that the doula was attempting to uphold. However, doulas were upfront about their belief that an unmedicated and nonintervention birth was preferred for the lower-risk woman, and this information in the form of education material was shared with clients in education classes and informal conversations:

> I like to use information from *Obstetric Myths Versus Research Realities* and work in as much current research as possible into my classes. In my experience there are care providers that are up on the most recent recommendations and those that haven't read research since med school. There are those providers that always do it one way and that doesn't work for every woman in birth so I want women to be well informed. (Megan, doula)

Doulas assert that their views on medication and intervention are consistent with current medical guidelines and recommendations, and that their intention is to share current knowledge with women that may or may not be well-informed by their care providers.

In comparison, women explained how the doula had to manage the woman's previous wishes when those wishes changed in labor and reflects a potential misassumption that doulas' have their own agenda:

> I told my doula and Peter that I wanted to do this naturally. I really wanted to try to go through labor and experience the birth. I think on some level I thought the pain was a rite of passage for me. I remember thinking that a natural birth was on the top of my list. That to be a good mother you had to have this traumatic painful birth and come out the other side a stronger better mother. Then of course during labor everything changes. I remember one point during a contraction I was begging for an epidural. At first I thought my doula was slow to respond. It seemed like it took such a long time to get the epidural and then once I got it the pain was gone but then I felt terrible. I remember crying a lot. My husband thought I was still in a lot of pain and so he went to find the nurse and then when he left I told our doula that I was so sorry and that I shouldn't have had the epidural and all this guilt just poured out of me. She just held me and said I made the right choice. She just kept saying, "You made the right choice." That really got

me through labor. Later, several days later, when we were talking she told me that my feelings were very normal. I told her that at first I was upset because I didn't feel like she wanted me to have an epidural. She said that it was difficult for her because she wanted to respect what I had in my birth plan but at the same time she thought that the epidural was a good choice. And I was like, you did? And she said, "Yes, you had gone so long without pain medication, working really hard and that was wonderful." She might have even said she was proud of me, but regardless, I felt like I was proud of myself. I hadn't felt that way about the birth before then. I think part of the guilt was saying that I would do it naturally and then not being able to, except that my doula reminded me that I went a long time without anything and then it was actually helpful in me getting some rest, since it had been a long labor, for the pushing stage. I think one of the most amazing things about my doula was her being able to be there to talk about my birth after my birth and help me think through all these emotions and some of the guilt I was carrying. (Amy, mother)

Amy, in her narrative, described how part of her guilt was a result of her feeling that her doula didn't "want her" to have the epidural. Amy may also be describing her own personal guilt of wanting an unmedicated birth but then changing her mind during labor. In labor, when Amy asked for pain relief, her doula's slowness to respond potentially represented the doula navigating a previous assertion—Amy's assertion of not wanting an epidural. As she talked through her birth with her doula, Amy was then surprised that her doula thought she made "the right choice." This represents an important perspective that other care providers may not understand: the doulas in filling the role of advocate must balance previous assertions given by their clients with in-the-moment changes during labor, but ultimately, doulas are there to support the woman's wishes and demonstrate both intimate care and personal advocacy.

Conclusion

Laura in the opening excerpt of this chapter stated that caring for a young pregnant teen, by modeling compassion and understanding of her experience during a transformative life transition such as childbirth, was modeling to women while in labor that they are loved. This is not to say that partners or family do not or cannot show their love and fill that caring role. The role of the doula is to model love in the physical and emotional support they offer while also remaining detached in order to advocate for the woman's wishes when necessary. For doulas, the reason women attain their own positive birth outcomes when birthing with a doula is because of the combination of love and advocacy by another woman, outside of the institutional domain and medical authoritarian model. Because of their philosophy of an *embodied* experience and their detached intimacy in the relationship, doulas can advocate for women in ways that family members may not be able to. Doulas hold the individual woman's personal agency and wishes about the birth experience as priority and her body as authority, which other care providers may not because of other institutional responsibilities or requirements.

While this book has lodged a critique that authoritative knowledge in the medicalization of childbirth has devalued women's experience and knowledge in birth, the same critique could be used to examine how the notion of "women's knowledge" has been understood from the perspective of a white middle-class woman. We do not know how women from different socioeconomic statuses or women of color perceive alternative models of health care and how their own cultural perceptions interact with alternative health education models. Nor do we know if there are differences in outcomes when there is a difference in class, race, ethnicity, or culture between the doula and her client.

It is also unrealistic to assume that all women have the choice to choose professional labor support. Childbirth education takes considerable time and monetary resources that are limited or unavailable to all women. Thus, the expectation of any care provider that childbirth education is universal makes both cultural and class assumptions. What has not been made explicit in medical literature is the variety of doula care that is available and how race, ethnicity, class, and culture have an impact on the choice of having a doula-assisted birth.

The current medical research does not recognize that women may have enough different experiences via culture, class, race, and ethnicity so that "any" doula cannot be a "universal" doula. The assumption of a "universal" doula comes from a privilege of whiteness that renders white as a "universal culture" without the reflection that those who are nonwhite do not have access to the "universal culture" in the same way. Likewise, "universalizing" the doula experience as an intervention for all women does not recognize the money and time needed to "prepare" for childbirth as well as the realization that an "educated contempt for professionals is less problematic for those who live among the educated as opposed to those who have to submit to experts in varied life experiences" (Nelson 1982, p. 295).

Race, ethnicity, class, and culture have not emerged as a significant topic in the scholarship on labor support women. If we assume that gender is always constructed in relation to race (Briggs 2000), then we must assume that the construction of childbirth as a gendered phenomenon has been likewise constructed as racially, class, and culturally defined. Much more research is needed to understand if what is presented in this book holds for women from different racial, ethnic, socioeconomic, or cultural groups. While the caution holds that universalizing any singular group's experience holds for all women, we do contend that an embodied experience in which the woman's body has privilege and support includes love and advocacy is beneficial to all women.

This book presents women's voices, doulas and mothers, working together to claim women's authority in body and in the birthing process. There are many things that this book could not completely express about the relationship between doulas and birthing women. Ultimately, the relationship between the doula and the woman that is created before, during, and after the birthing experience can never be fully articulated. We will conclude with two comments, one from a birthing woman participant and one from a doula. The attempt is to close with a final endeavor at articulating what resides in the relationship between doulas and birthing women, in their own words:

> I remember when I was birthing on my hands and knees and I just knew she was back there. But then at one moment I just remember having a feeling of panic that I couldn't, that she wasn't touching me anywhere. I remember being a bit scared thinking where is she, and so I just remember saying, "Are you there, are you there, are you there?" And then she just put her hand on my back. And I was like, "I'm okay." (Lisa, mother)
>
> I play the role of witnessing and remembering for the woman, and holding the space so that it unfolds. The strength is there in the woman, it is not something I give to her. I just support her on her journey to find it. And I want to be there for her if she doesn't see it. Sometimes women think they can't or aren't doing very well in labor and I point out how, at that particular moment, how amazing she is, that she *is* (emphasis added) doing it. (Jennifer, doula)

References

Adams, E., & Bianchi, A. L. (2008). A practical approach to labor support. *Journal of Obstetric, Gynecologic, and Neonatal Nursing, 37*, 106–111.

American Association of University Women. (2001). "Hostile hallways: Bullying, teasing, and sexual harassment in school". In UN General Assembly (2006), *In-depth study on all forms of violence against women: Report of the secretary-general*, A/61/122/Add.1, p. 42, New York. Retrieved from http://www.unwomen.org/en/what-we-do/ending-violence-against-women/facts-and-figures#sthash.CIe0BhG6.dpuf

American College of Obstetricians and Gynecologists. (2006). *ACOG recommends restricted use of episiotomies*. Washington, DC: American College of Obstetricians and Gynecologists.

American College of Obstetricians and Gynecologists. (2009). ACOG Practice Bulletin No. 106: Intrapartum fetal heart rate monitoring: Nomenclature, interpretation, and general management principles. *Obstetrics and Gynecology, 114*(1), 192.

American Council of Obstetrics and Gynecology. (2014). *Re: Methods for estimating due dates*. Retrieved from http://www.acog.org/Resources-And-Publications/Committee-Opinions/Committee-on-Obstetric-Practice/Method-for-Estimating-Due-Date

Amram, N. L., Klein, M. C., Mok, H., Simkin, P., Lindstrom, K., & Grant, J. (2014). How birth doulas help clients adapt to changes in circumstances, clinical care, and client preferences during labor. *The Journal of Perinatal Education, 23*(2), 96–103. doi:10.1891/1058-1243.23.2.96.

Anderson, C. J., & Kilpatrick, C. (2012). Supporting patients' birth plans: Theories, strategies and implications for nurses. *Nursing for Women's Health, 16*(3), 210–218. doi:10.1111/j.1751-486X.2012.01732.x

Ashford, J. (1998). *The timeless way: A history of birth from ancient to modern times [videotape]*. Boulder: Injoy Videos.

Bäckström, C., & Hertfelt Wahn, E. (2011). Support during labour: First-time fathers' descriptions of requested and received support during the birth of their child. *Midwifery, 27*(1), 67–73. doi:10.1016/j.midw.2009.07.001.

Bailit, J. L., Gregory, K. D., Reddy, U. M., Gonzalez-Quintero, V. H., Hibbard, J. U., Ramirez, M. M., ... Zhang, J. (2010). Maternal and neonatal outcomes by labor onset type and gestational age. *American Journal of Obstetrics and Gynecology, 202*(3), 245.e1. http://dx.doi.org/10.1016/j.ajog.2010.01.051

Barker, P. M., & Olver, R. E. (2002). Invited review: Clearance of lung liquid during the perinatal period. *Journal of Applied Physiology, 93*(4), 1542–1548. doi:10.1152/japplphysiol.00092.2002.

Barry, H., & Paxson, L. M. (1971). Infancy and early childhood: Cross-cultural codes. *Ethnology, 10*, 466–508.

Berg, C. J., Callaghan, W. M., Syverson, C., & Henderson, Z. (2010). Pregnancy-related mortality in the United States, 1998 to 2005. *Obstetrics and Gynecology, 116*(6), 1302–1309. doi:10.1097/AOG.0b013e3181fdfb11.

Bertsch, T. D., Nagashima-Whalen, L., Dykeman, S., Kennell, J. H., & McGrath, S. K. (1990). Labor support by first-time fathers: Direct observations. *Journal of Psychosomatic Obstetrics and Gynaeology, 11*, 251–260.

Birth Stories. (2007). *Re: Epidural Man [weblog]*. Retrieved from http://www.birthstories.com/stories/2643.php?wcat=35

Birth Stories. (2010). *Re: Touch of a Doula [web blog]*. Retrieved from http://lironsharon.com/Birth-Stories.php

Birth Without Fear. (2013). *Re: The difference a doula makes[web blog]*. Retrieved from http://birthwithoutfearblog.com/2013/01/05/the-difference-a-doula-makes-a-birth-story/

Blackwell, B. (2001). Tristam Shandy and the theater of the mechanical mother. *English Library History, 68*(1), 81–133.

Blanton, W. B. (1972). *Medicine in Virginia in the seventeenth century*. New York: Arno Press. reprint.

Bogdan, J. (1978). Care or cure? Childbirth practices in nineteenth century America. *Feminist Studies, 4*(2), 92–99.

Bourgeault, I. L., & Fynes, M. (1997). Integrating lay and nurse-midwifery into the U.S. and Canadian healthcare systems. *Social Science and Medicine, 44*(7), 1051–1063.

Briggs, L. (2000). The race of hysteria: Overcivilization and the savage woman in late nineteenth-century obstetrics and gynecology. *American Quarterly, 52*(2), 246–273.

Brooks, A. K., Kennell, J. H., & McGrath, S. K. (1995). Supportive behaviors of men and women during labor. *Pediatric Research, 37*, 13A.

Bulletin of the lying-in hospital of the city of New York (1913) Volumes 8–9. New York (N.Y.) Lying-in Hospital.

Bureau of Justice Statistics. (2012) *Re: Press release: Nearly 3.4 million violent cries per year went unreported to police from 2006 to 2010.* Retrieved from http://www.bjs.gov/content/pub/press/vnrp0610pr.cfm

Burrows, L. J., Meyn, L. A., & Weber, A. M. (2004). Maternal morbidity associated with vaginal versus cesarean delivery. *Obstetrics and Gynecology, 103,* 907–912.

Camann, W. (2014). A history of pain relief during childbirth. In *The wondrous story of anesthesia* (pp. 847–858). New York: Springer.

Carspecken, P. F. (2001). *Critical ethnography in education.* New York: Routledge.

Caton, D. (1999). *What a blessing she had chloroform: The medical and social response to the pain of childbirth from 1800 to the present.* New Haven: Yale University Press.

Caughey, A. B., Cahill, A. G., Guise, J. M., Rouse, D. J., & American College of Obstetricians and Gynecologists. (2014). Safe prevention of the primary cesarean delivery. *American Journal of Obstetrics and Gynecology, 210*(3), 179–193.

Center for Disease Control. (2013). *Re: Births – method of delivery.* Retrieved from http://www.cdc.gov/nchs/fastats/delivery.htm

Center for Disease Control. (2014). *Re: Preterm birth [Web log post].* Retrieved from http://www.cdc.gov/reproductivehealth/maternalinfanthealth/pretermbirth.htm

Chmell, A. (2012). Home sweet home. A place to deliver, care for, and raise our children. *The Journal of Legal Medicine, 33,* 137–148. doi:10.1080/01947648.2012.657949.

Cobb, S. (1976). Social support as a moderator of life stress. *Psychosomatic Medicine, 38*(5), 300–314.

Code, L. (1991). *What can she know? Feminist theory and the construction of knowledge.* Ithaca: Cornell University Press.

Colligan, L., Potts, H. W., Finn, C. T., & Sinkin, R. A. (2015). Cognitive workload changes for nurses transitioning from a legacy system with paper documentation to a commercial electronic health record. *International Journal of Medical Informatics, 84*(7), 469–476.

Conrad, P. (1992). Medicalization and social-control. *Annual Review of Sociology, 18,* 209–232.

Cornell, D. (1998). *At the heart of freedom.* Princeton: Princeton University Press.

Craven, C. (2005). Claiming respectable American motherhood: Homebirth mothers, medical officials, and the state. *Medical Anthropology Quarterly, 19*(2), 194–215.

Cutrona, G. E., & Russell, D. W. (1990). Type of social support and specific stress: Toward a theory of optimal matching. In I. G. Sarason, B. R. Sarason, & G. R. Pierce (Eds.), *Social support and interactional view* (pp. 319–366). New York: John Wiley & Sons.

Cutter, I. S., & Viets, H. R. (1964). *A short history of midwifery.* Philadelphia: Saunders.

Davis-Floyd, R. E. (1992). *Birth as an American right of passage*. Berkeley: University of California Press.
Declercq, E., Barger, M., Cabral, H. J., Evans, S. R., Kotelchuck, M., Simon, C., ... Heffner, L. J. (2007). Maternal outcomes associated with planned primary cesarean births compared with planned vaginal births. *Obstetrics and Gynecology, 109*(3), 669–677. http://dx.doi.org/10.1097/01.AOG.0000255668.20639.40
Dekker, R. (2013). *National birth center study II*. American Association of Birth Centers. Retrieved from http://www.birthcenters.org/?page=NBCSII
Delay, T., Kennell, J. H., & Klaus, M. (1987). Supportive companions of women in labor: A descriptive analysis. *Pediatric Research, 6*, 61.
Department of Health. (2004). *National service framework for children, young people and maternity services*. Retrieved from https://www.gov.uk/government/uploads/system/uploads/attachment_data/file/199952/National_Service_Framework_for_Children_Young_People_and_Maternity_Services_Core_Standards.pdf
Dick-Read, G. (1933). *Natural childbirth*. London: Heinemann.
Dick-Read, G. (1960). *Childbirth without fear*. London: Heinemann.
DONA International. (2005). *What is a doula?* Retrieved from http://www.dona.org/mothers/index.php
DTI Admin. (2013). *Re: Holding the space [Web log post]*. Retrieved from http://www.doulatraininginternational.com/holding-the-space
Durkheim, E. (1951). *Suicide: A study in sociology* (trans: Simpson, J. A. S. G.). Illinois: Glencoe Press.
Eftekhary, S., Klein, M. C., & Xu, S. Y. (2010). The life of a Canadian doula: Successes, confusion, and conflict. *Journal of Obstetrics and Gynaecology Canada, 32*(7), 642–649.
Elbourne, D., Oakley, A., & Chalmers, I. (1989). Social and psychological support during pregnancy. In I. Chalmers, M. Enkin, & M. Keirse (Eds.), *Effective care in pregnancy and childbirth* (Vol. 1). Oxford: Oxford University Press.
Faxelius, G., Hägnevik, K., Lagercrantz, H., Lundell, B., & Irestedt, L. (1983). Catecholamine surge and lung function after delivery. *Archives of Disease in Childhood, 58*(4), 262–266.
Fitzgerald v. Porter Memorial. 523 F. 2d 716 (7th Cir. 1975).
Gadamer, H. G. (2004). *Truth and method* (trans: Weinsheimer, J. & Marshall, D. G. 2nd Ed.). New York: Continuum.
Gagnon, A. J., & Waghorn, K. (1996). Supportive care by maternity nurses: A work sampling study in an intrapartum unit. *Birth (Berkeley, Calif.), 23*(1), 1–6.
Gilliland, A. L. (2011). After praise and encouragement: Emotional support strategies used by birth doulas in the USA and Canada. *Midwifery, 27*(4), 525–531. doi:10.1016/j.midw.2010.04.006.
Goer, H. (1995). *Obstetric myths and research realities: A guide to the medical literature*. Westport, CT: Bergin & Garvey Publishers.

Goer, H., & Romano, A. M. (2012). *Optimal care in childbirth: The case for a physiologic approach.* Seattle: Classic Day Publishing. Retrieved from http://www.optimalcareinchildbirth.com/

Gordon, N., Walton, D., McAdam, E., Deman, J., & Gallitero, G. (1999). Effects of providing hospital-based doulas in health maintenance organization hospitals. *Obstetrics and Gynecology, 93*(3), 422–426.

Gottlieb, B. H. (1981). Development and application of a classification scheme of informal helping behaviour. *Canadian Journal of Behavioral Science, 10,* 105–115.

Grosz, E. (1994). *Volatile bodies: Toward a corporeal feminism.* Bloomington: Indiana University Press.

Gruber, K. J., Cupito, S. H., & Dobson, C. F. (2013). Impact of doulas on healthy birth outcomes. *The Journal of Perinatal Education, 22*(1), 49. doi:10.1891/1058-1243.22.1.49.

Gurevich, R. (2003). *The doula advantage.* Roseville: Random House.

Hartmann, K., Viswanathan, M., Palmieri, R., Gartlehner, G., Thorp, J., & Lohr, K. N. (2005). Outcomes of routine episiotomy: A systematic review. *Jama, 293*(17), 2141–2148. doi:10.1001/jama.293.17.2141.

Henderson, J., & Redshaw, M. (2013). Who is well after childbirth? Factors related to positive outcome. *Birth, 40*(1), 1–9. doi:10.1111/birt.12022.

Hendrich, A., Chow, M. P., Skierczynski, B. A., & Lu, Z. (2008). A 36-hospital time and motion study: How do medical-surgical nurses spend their time? *The Permanente Journal, 12*(3), 25.

Hikel, K. (2009). *Autism, ADHD, and medicated births.* Medscape multispecialty. 28 May 2009 Retrieved from http://www.medscape.com/viewarticle/703211_2

Hodnett, E. D., Gates, S., Hofmeyr, G.J., & Sakala, C. (2012). Continuous support for women during childbirth. *Cochrane Database of Systematic Reviews,* Issue 10. Art. No.: CD003766. http://dx.doi.org/10.1002/14651858.CD003766.pub4

Hofmeyer, G. J., Nikodem, V. C., Wolman, W. L., Chalmers, B. E., & Kramer, T. (1991). Companionship to modify the clinical birth environment: Effects on progress and perceptions of labor and breast feeding. *British Journal of Obstetrics and Gynaecology, 98*(8), 756–764.

Howarth, A., Swain, N., & Treharne, G. J. (2011). Taking personal responsibility for well-being increases birth satisfaction of first time mothers. *Journal of Health Psychology, 16,* 1221–1230. doi:10.1177/1359105311403521.

Howell-White, S. (1999). Choosing a birth attendant: The influences of a women's childbirth definition. *Social Science and Medicine, 45,* 925–936.

ICEA. (1999). ICEA position paper: The role and scope of the doula. *International Journal of Childbirth Education Association, 14,* 38–45.

Informed Medical Decisions Foundation. (2015). *What is shared decision making?* Retrieved from http://www.informedmedicaldecisions.org/what-is-shared-decision-making/

Jansen, L., Gibson, M., Bowles, B. C., & Leach, J. (2013). First do no harm: Interventions during childbirth. *The Journal of Perinatal Education, 22*(2), 83–92. doi:10.1891/1058-1243.22.2.83.

Johanson, R., Newburn, M., & Macfarlane, A. (2002). Has the medicalisation of childbirth gone too far? *British Medical Journal, 324*(7342), 892–895. doi:10.1136/bmj.324.7342.892.

Johnson, M. P. (2002). The implications of unfulfilled expectations and perceived pressure to attend the birth on men's stress levels following birth attendance: A longitudinal study. *Journal of Psychosomatic Obstetrics and Gynecology, 23*(3), 173–182.

Jordan, B. (1997). Authoritative knowledge and its construction. In R. E. Davis-Floyd & C. F. Sargent (Eds.), *Childbirth and authoritative knowledge*. Berkeley: University of California Press.

Kahn, R. L., & Antonucci, T. C. (1980). Convoys over the life course: Attachment roles and social support. In P. B. Baltes & O. Brim (Eds.), *Life span development and behavior* (pp. 253–286). New York: Academic.

Kayne, M. A., Greulich, M. B., & Albers, L. L. (2001). Doulas: An alternative yet complementary addition to care during childbirth. *Clinical Obstetrics and Gynecology, 44*(4), 692–703.

Kennell, J. H. (2004). Benefits of a doula present at the birth of a child. *Pediatrics, 114*(5), 1489.

Kennell, J. H., Klaus, M. H., McGrath, S. K., Robertson, S. S., & Hinkley, C. W. (1991). Continuous emotional support during labor in a US hospital. *Journal of the American Medical Association, 265*, 2197–2201.

Ketler, S. (2000). Preparing for motherhood: Authoritative knowledge and the undercurrents of shared experience in two childbirth education courses in Cagliari, Italy. *Medical Anthropology Quarterly, 14*(2), 138–158.

Kilpatrick, Dean G., Ph.D., Heidi S. Resnick, Ph.D., Kenneth J. Ruggiero, Ph.D., Lauren M. Conoscenti, M. A., & Jenna McCauley, M. S. (2011). *Re: Drug-Facilitated, incapacitated, and forcible rape: A national study*. Retrieved from https://www.ncjrs.gov/pdffiles1/nij/grants/219181.pdf

Kitzinger, S. (1997). Authoritative touch in childbirth. In R. E. Davis-Floyd & C. F. Sargent (Eds.), *Childbirth and authoritative knowledge*. Berkeley: University of California Press.

Klaus, M., & Klaus, P. (2010). Academy of breastfeeding medicine founder's lecture: Maternity care re-evaluated. *Breastfeeding Medicine, 5*(1), 3–8.

Klaus, M. H., Kennell, J. H., Robertson, S. S., & Sosa, R. (1986). Effects of social support during parturition on maternal and infant morbity. *British Medical Journal, 293*, 585–587.

Kobayashi, H., Reid, G., & Hadfield, M. (2014). Effects of vaginal delivery, cesarean section and exposure to labor on endothelial function of pregnant women. *Thrombosis Research, 134*(5), 1004–1007.

Kozak, L. J., Owings, M. F., & Hall, M. J. (2004). National hospital discharge survey: 2001 annual summary with detailed diagnosis and procedure data. *Vital Health Statistics, 13*(156), 1–198.

Lally, J. E., Thomson, R. G., MacPhail, S., & Exley, C. (2014). Pain relief in labour: A qualitative study to determine how to support women to make decisions about pain relief in labour. *BMC Pregnancy and Childbirth, 14*(1), 6.

Lamaze, F. (1956). *Painless childbirth: The lamaze method* (trans: Celestin, L. R.). Chicago: Contemporary Books.

Leavitt, J. W. (1980). Birthing and Anesthesia: The debate over twilight sleep. *Signs: Journal of Women in Culture and Society, 6*(1).

Lee, H. C., Gould, J. B., Boscardin, W. J., El-Sayed, Y. Y., & Blumenfeld, Y. J. (2011). Trends in cesarean delivery for twin births in the United States: 1995 to 2008. *Obstetrics and Gynecology, 118*(5), 1095.

Lefcourt, H. M. (1984). *Research with the locus of control construct* (Vol. 2). New York: Academic.

Little, S. E., Edlow, A. G., Thomas, A. M., & Smith, N. A. (2012). Estimated fetal weight by ultrasound: A modifiable risk factor for cesarean delivery? *American Journal of Obstetrics and Gynecology, 207*(4), 309.e1.

Lothian, J. A. (2006). Saying "no" to induction. *The Journal of Perinatal Education, 15*(2), 43–45. doi:10.1624/105812406X107816.

Loudon, I. (1992). *Death in childbirth: An international study of maternal care and maternal mortality 1800–1950*. Oxford: Clarendon.

MacDorman, M. F., Declercq, E., & Menacker, F. (2011). Trends and characteristics of home births in the United States by race and ethnicity, 1990–2006. *Birth, 38*(1), 17–23. doi:10.1111/j.1523-536X.2010.00444.

MacDorman, M. F., Mathews, T. J., & Declercq, E. R. (2012). *Home births in the United States,1990–2009*. US Department of Health and Human Services, Centers for Disease Control and Prevention, National Center for Health Statistics. Retrieved from http://dhmh.md.gov/midwives/Documents/Declercq-2009-HBdatabrief.pdf

Madden, K. L., Turnbull, D., Cyna, A. M., Adelson, P., & Wilkinson, C. (2013). Pain relief for childbirth: The preferences of pregnant women, midwives and obstetricians. *Women and Birth, 26*(1), 33–40.

Madi, B. C., Sandall, J., Bennett, R., & Macleod, C. (1999). Effects of female relative support in labor: A randomized controlled trial. *Birth: Issues in Perinatal Care, 26*(1), 4–8.

Malacrida, C., & Boulton, T. (2013). The best laid plans? Women's choices, expectations and experiences in childbirth. *Health, 18*, 41–59. 1363459313476964.

Mander, R. (2001). *Supportive care and midwifery*. Oxford: Blackwell Science Ltd.

Martens, P. J. (2000). Does breastfeeding education affect nursing staff beliefs, exclusive breastfeeding rates, and baby-friendly hospital initiative compliance?

The experience of a small, rural Canadian hospital. *Journal of Human Lactation, 16*(4), 309–318. doi:10.1177/089033440001600407.

Martin, J. A., Hamilton, B. E., Ventura, S. J., Osterman, M. J., Kirmeyer, S., Mathews, T. J., & Wilson, E. C. (2009). Births: Final data for 2009. *National Vital Statistics Reports: From the Centers for Disease Control and Prevention, National Center for Health Statistics, National Vital Statistics System, 60*(1), 1–70.

Marx, K. (1983). *The portable Karl Marx*. New York: Penguin Press.

Mayo Clinic. (2015). *Re: Inducing labor*. Retrieved from http://www.mayoclinic.org/healthy-lifestyle/labor-and-delivery/in-depth/inducing-labor/art-20047557

Meyer, B., Arnold, J., & Pascali-Bonaro, D. (2001). Social support by doulas during labor and the early postpartum period. *Hospital Physician, 37*, 57–65.

Miller, K., & Ray, E. B. (1994). Beyond the ties that bind us: Exploring the meaning of supportive messages and relationships. In B. R. Barleson, T. L. Albrecht, & I. G. Sarason (Eds.), *Communication of social support* (pp. 215–228). London: Sage.

Morton, C. H. (2002). *Doula care: The (Re)emergence of woman supported childbirth in the United States*. Los Angeles: University of California.

Munro, S., Kornelsen, J., & Grzybowski, S. (2013). Models of maternity care in rural environments: Barriers and attributes of interprofessional collaboration with midwives. *Midwifery, 29*(6), 646–652. doi:10.1016/j.midw.2012.06.004.

Nelson, M. (1982). The effect of childbirth preparation on women of different social classes. *Journal of Health and Social Behavior, 23*, 339–352.

O'Brian, M. (1995). Reproducing Marxist man. In N. Tuana & R. Tong (Eds.), *Feminism and philosophy: Essential readings in theory, reinterpretation, and application*. Boulder: Westview Press.

Ophir, E., Strulov, A., Solt, I., Michlin, R., Buryanov, I., & Bornstein, J. (2008). Delivery mode and maternal rehospitalization. *Archives of Gynecology and Obstetrics, 277*(5), 401–404. doi:10.1007/s00404-007-0476-4.

Papagni, K., & Buckner, E. (2006). Doula support and attitudes of intrapartum nurses: A qualitative study from the patient's perspective. *The Journal of Perinatal Education, 15*(1), 11. doi:10.1624/105812406X92949.

Pascali-Bonaro, D. (2003). Childbirth education and doula care during times of stress; trauma, and grieving. *The Journal of Perinatal Education, 12*(4), 1–7.

Pfuntner, A., Wier, L. M., & Stocks, C. (2013). *Most frequent procedures performed in US Hospitals, 2011*.

PHDOULA. (2009). *Re: My first birth: a doula's-eye birth story*. Retrieved from http://dynamicdoula.blogspot.com/2009/10/my-first-birth-doulas-eye-birth-story.html

Phillips, C. R. (2003). *Family-centered maternity care*. Burlington: Jones & Bartlett Learning.

Regan, M., McElroy, K. G., & Moore, K. (2013). Choice? Factors that influence women's decision making for childbirth. *The Journal of Perinatal Education, 22*(3), 171–180. doi:10.1891/1058-1243.22.3.171.

Richmond Doulas. (2012). *Re: Heather M.'s birth story [web blog]*. Retrieved from http://www.richmonddoulas.org/blog/for-moms-4/birth-stories/heather-m-s-birth-story/

Robson, C. (2002). *Real world research*. Sussex: Wiley.

Salminen, S., Gibson, G. R., McCartney, A. L., & Isolauri, E. (2004). Influence of mode of delivery on gut microbiota composition in seven year old children. *Gut, 53*(9), 1388–1389. doi:10.1136/gut.2004.041640.

Sapountzi-Krepia, D., Psychogiou, M., Sakellari, E., Tsiligiri, M., & Vehvilainen-Julkunen, K. (2014). Greek fathers' experiences from their wife's/partner's labour and delivery: A qualitative approach. *International Journal of Nursing Practice, 21*, 470–477. doi:10.1111/ijn.12326.

Sarason, I. G., Sarason, B. R., & Pierce, G. R. (1990). Relationship specific social support: Towards a model for the analysis of supportive interactions. In B. R. Barleson, T. L. Albrecht, & I. G. Sarason (Eds.), *Communication and social support* (p. 91). London: Sage.

Say, R., Robson, S., & Thomson, R. (2011). Helping pregnant women make better decisions: A systematic review of the benefits of patient decision aids in obstetrics. *British Medical Journal Open, 1*(2), e000261. doi:10.1136/bmjopen-2011-000261.

Scott, K. D., Berkowitz, G., & Klaus, M. H. (1999). A comparison of intermittent and continuous support during labor: A meta-analysis. *American Journal of Obstetrics and Gynecology, 180*, 1054.

Sheffield, J. S., Hollier, L. M., Hill, J. B., Stuart, G. S., & Wendel, G. D. (2003). Acyclovir prophylaxis to prevent herpes simplex virus recurrence at delivery: A systematic review. *Obstetrics and Gynecology, 102*(6), 1396–1403. doi:10.1016/j.obstetgynecol.2003.08.015.

Simkin, P. (1991). Just another day in a woman's life? Part II: Nature and consistency of women's long-term memories of their first birth experiences. *Birth, 19*(2), 64–81.

Simkin, P. (1992). The labor support person: Latest addition to the maternity care team? *International Journal of Childbirth Education, 7*(1), 19–24.

Simkin, P. (2005). Why keep on keeping on? *Journal of Perinatal Education, 14*(2), 5–7.

Sleutel, M., Schultz, S., & Wyble, K. (2007). Nurses' views of factors that help and hinder their intrapartum care. *Journal of Obstetric, Gynecologic, and Neonatal Nursing, 36*(3), 203–211.

Smid, M., Campero, L., Cragin, L., Hernandez, D. G., & Walker, D. (2010). Bringing two worlds together: Exploring the integration of traditional mid-

wives as doulas in Mexican public hospitals. *Health Care for Women International, 31*(6), 475–498. doi:10.1080/07399331003628438.
Smith, A. C. (2011). Role ambiguity and role conflict in nurse case managers: An integrative review. *Professional Case Management, 16*(4), 182–196. doi:10.1097/NCM.0b013e318218845b.
Smyth, S., Spence, D., & Murray, K. (2015). Does antenatal education prepare fathers for their role as birth partners and for parenthood? *British Journal of Midwifery, 23*(5), 336–342.
Sosa, R., Kennell, J. H., Klaus, M. H., Robertson, S., & Urrutia, J. (1980). The effect of a supportive companion on perinatal problems, length of labor, and mother-infant interaction. *The New England Journal of Medicine, 303*(11), 597–600.
Spiby, H., Henderson, B., Slade, P., Escott, D., Fraser, R. B., & Spiby, H. (1999). Strategies for coping with labour: Does antenatal education translate into practice? *Journal of Advanced Nursing, 29*(2), 388–395.
Spitzer, A., Bar-Tal, Y., & Golander, H. (1995). Social support: How does it really work? *Journal of Advanced Nursing, 22*, 850–854.
Tarkka, M., & Paunonen, M. (1996). Social support and its impact on mothers' experiences of childbirth. *Journal of Advanced Nursing, 23*, 70–75.
Thacker, S. B., Stroup, D. F., & Peterson, H. B. (1995). Efficacy and safety of intrapartum electronic fetal monitoring: An update. *Obstetrics and Gynecology, 86*(4), 613–620. doi:10.1016/S0029-7844(95)80027-1.
Thoits, P. A. (1982). Life stress, social support, and psychological vulnerability: Epidemiological considerations. *Journal of Community Psychology, 10*, 341–362.
Tong, R. (1989). *Feminist thought: A comprehensive introduction.* Boulder: Westview Press.
UNICEF. (2015). *The baby-friendly hospital initiative.* Retrieved from http://www.unicef.org/programme/breastfeeding/baby.htm
van Teijlingen, E., Wrede, S., Benoit, C., Sandall, J., & DeVries, R. (2009). Born in the USA: Exceptionalism in maternity care organisation among high-income countries. *Sociological Research Online, 14*(1), 5. doi:10.5153/sro.1860.
Waldenstrom, U. (2004). Why do some women change their opinion about childbirth over time? *Birth, 31*(2), 102–107.
Walker, D. S., Visger, J. M., & Rossie, D. (2009). Contemporary childbirth education models. *Journal of Midwifery and Women's Health, 54*(6), 469–476. doi:10.1016/j.jmwh.2009.02.013.
Walling, A. D. (2002, November 15). Epidural analgesia prolongs the active phase of labor. *American Family Physician.* Available at: http://www.aafp.org/afp/20021115/tips/18.html. Accessed 12 Mar 2009.
Webb, D. A., & Robbins, J. M. (2003). Mode of delivery and risk of postpartum rehospitalization. *Journal of the American Medical Association, 289*(46), 7.
Wertz, D. C. (1996). What birth has done for doctors. In P. K. Wilson (Ed.), *Childbirth: Changing ideas and practices in Britain and America 1600 to the present* (Vol. 2, pp. 3–20). New York: Garland Publishing.

Wertz, R. W., & Wertz, D. C. (1989). *Lying-in: A history of childbirth in America*. New Haven: Yale University Press.

Wheatley, S. (1998). Psychosocial support in pregnancy. In S. Clement (Ed.), *Psychological perspectives on pregnancy and childbirth* (pp. 45–59). Edinburgh: Churchill Livingstone.

Wolman, W. L. (1991). *Social support during childbirth: Psychological and physiological outcomes*. Johannesburg: University of Witwatersand.

World Health Organization. (1996). *Care in normal birth: A practical guide*. Geneva: Department of reproductive health and research. World Health Organization.

World Health Organization. (2011). *WHO recommendations for induction of labour*. Geneva: World Health Organization.

Young, I. M. (1995). Pregnant embodiment: Subjectivity and alienation. In N. Tuana & R. Tong (Eds.), *Feminism and philosophy: Essential readings in theory, reinterpretation, and application*. Boulder: Westview Press.

Zhang, J., Bernasko, J. W., Leybovich, E., Fahs, M., & Hatch, M. C. (1996). Continuous labor support from labor attendant for primaparous women: A meta-analysis. *Obstetrics and Gynecology, 88*(4), 739–744.

INDEX

A
advocacy, 116, 124
  caregiving role, 113
  detached caring, 117–22
  physical and emotional support, 115
alienation and authority
  in American medical context, 58
  authoritative knowledge system, 54
  death rates, childbirth, 61
  Engels's theory, 55
  "epidural man", 60–1
  epidural use and cesarean sections, 52–3
  healthy birthing women, 58
  hospital-based class, 53
  hospital protocols, 52
  labor of childbirth, 55
  language, 53
  medical model, 51
  medical professional, 59
  waiting for labor, 55–6
  web blog, 60–1
alternative knowledge systems, 61
American birthing practices, 4–5, 76
American Council of Obstetrics and Gynecology (ACOG), 6, 7, 77

American Journal of Obstetrics, 66
antenatal classes, 32–3, 38, 43
authoritative knowledge, 54
  medical institution, 62
  medical knowledge, 63–4

B
baby-friendly hospital policies, 29
birthing event, 72, 78–9, 84, 105
birthing women, 15, 19, 55, 58, 66, 72, 80, 82, 110, 124
birth plan, 9, 23, 29, 41, 44, 114, 117, 118
blood–brain barrier, 5
breast-feeding, 3, 10, 13, 14, 28, 29, 44, 72, 88, 89

C
"catching", 88
catecholamines, 7
Centers for Disease Control and Prevention (CDC), 59, 77
Cesarean section, 53, 58
  ACOG, 8

Cesarean section (*cont.*)
  catecholamines, 7
  depressed immune system, 8
  gastrointestinal tract, 8
  thoracic cage, 7
childbirth as pathological
  counterdiscourse on doulas, 69–71
  midwifery, 65
  natural childbirth movement, 66
  obstetrician-attended births, 65
  pathological agency, 67–9
Childbirth Without Fear (Dick-Read), 68
clinical dating methods, 77
colostrum, 88
continual moment, 81
contractions, timing of, 81–2

D
"delivering", 31, 56, 59, 68, 75, 76, 88
depressed immune system, 8
detached caring, 122
  caregiver, 118–19
  labor support, 118
  level of care doulas, 117
  medication and intervention, 121
  pain control, 120
DONA International, 2–3
doula–mother relationship, 109–10
doulas (labor support women)
  birth center/home birth, 46–7
  birth plan, 44
  DONA, 2
  educational and emotional support, 44
  as educator, 3
  meta-analysis, 11
  mother–infant bonding, 10
  obstetricians and nurses, 43
  parents space, 47
  physical and emotional support, 3
  postpartum period, 12
  role, 3–4

  and women, relationship, 13
  birthing women, 15
  childbirth education, 16
  ethnographic data, 20–1
  organization materials, 15
  participants, 14, 18–19
  postsecondary education, 17–18
  primary childbirth organization, 14–15
  transformative birth experiences, 21–4

E
elective induction, 5
electronic fetal monitoring (EFM), 5, 6
electronic health records (EHRs), 27
embodied language, 88–92. *See also* language, embodied
embodied space, birth, 85. *See also* experience, embodied
embodied time, birth, 75–6. *See also* time, embodied
emotional support, 31
  antenatal classes, 43
  pain, 42
  productive pain, 41
  Twilight Birth, 41
  uncertainty and frustration, 43
Engels's theory, 55
episiotomy, 6–7, 45, 99, 117
experience, embodied, 85
  erlebnis (experiential and embodied birth), 86
  hospital, 86–7
  language, challenge, 87

F
Family-Centered Maternity Care, 31–2
female support, 39

G
gastrointestinal tract, 8

H
"holding the space", 74
home births, 39, 59

I
intimacy, one-sided, 108, 113

L
Lamaze method, 31, 32, 40, 68
language, embodied, 89
  breast-feeding, 88
  catching and delivering, 88
  colostrum, 88
  labor process, 91
  nonverbal, 90
  vocalizations, 92
love
  and advocacy
    post-partum depression, 100
    socioemotional support, 102–6
  doula–woman relationship, 107
  intimacy, 108, 113
  mothering, 112
  physical support techniques, 110

M
medical interventions
  blood–brain barrier, 5
  cesarean section, 7–9
  EFM, 6
  elective induction, 5
  episiotomy, 6–7
  oxytocin, 5
midwifery, 15–16, 38, 59, 65, 76, 80, 101
mother–infant bonding, 10, 12
'mothering the mother', 109–10

N
national crime statistics, 94
Natural Childbirth (Dick-Read), 14, 22, 45, 68
natural childbirth movement, 66
nursing support
  baby-friendly hospital policies, 29
  EHRs, 27
  labor support, 25–6
  medicalization, childbirth, 26
  medical technology and electronic charting, 28
  obstetric nurses, 26
  women and nurses, 27

O
Obstetric Myths Versus Research Realities (Goer), 77
oxytocin, 5, 26

P
parents space, 47
partner and family support
  ambiguity (*see* (role ambiguity))
  antenatal classes, 32–3
  anxiety, 36
  decision-making process, 35–6
  emotional support (*see* (emotional support))
  Family-Centered Maternity Care, 31–2
  female support, 39
  home births, 39
  Lamaze method, 31
pathological agency, 67–9
physical support techniques, 110
Pitocin®, 60
post-partum
  depression, 100
  labour, 12
Productive pain, 41, 43

R

role ambiguity
  childbirth, 36
  communication, care providers and patients, 37
  negative perception, 38
  participation in labor, 36–7
  and stress, 38

S

scientific scripts
  clinical dating methods, 77
  compliance, notion of, 76
  due dates, 78
  time and haste, 76–7
shared decision-making, 10
  data analysis, 9
  labor and delivery, 9
socioemotional support
  childbirth experience, 106
  emotional support, 105
  father's support, 103
  interpersonal relationships, 102
  postpartum depression, 104

T

The Female Physician,.. The Whole Art of New Improved Midwifery (Maubray), 76
thoracic cage, 7
time, embodied
  birthing event, 78–9
  birth time, 80–1
  bodily signs, 84–5
  continual moment, 81
  contractions, 81–2
  distraction, 82
  embodied experience, 85–7
  embodied language, 88–92
  embodied space and process, 75, 85
  mechanical time, 83–4
  role, childbirth, 74
  scientific scripts, childbirth, 76–8
  space, holding, 74 (*see also* woman's body, understanding)
transformative birth experiences, 21–4
Twilight Birth, concept of, 41
Twilight Sleep movement, 67

V

vocalizations, 58, 84, 91, 92

W

web blog birth experience, 61
woman's body, understanding
  birth process, 95–6
  and bodily knowledge, labor, 58
  childbirth and breast-feeding, 89
  doula-led experience, 2
  embodied signals, 96
  female *vs.* male obstetrician/gynecologist, 93
  labor process, 91
  labor support, 92–3
  national crime statistics, 94

CPSIA information can be obtained
at www.ICGtesting.com
Printed in the USA
LVOW13*2236081017
551683LV00010BA/702/P